PAIN
Solutions

A Lee Dellon, MD, PhD, FACS

Director of the Dellon Institutes for Peripheral Nerve Surgery®

PUBLISHED BY

Lightning Source Inc
1246 Heil Quaker Blvd
La Vergne, TN 37086
USA
615 213 5815 / www.lightningsource.com

ISBN — 978-1-60402-697-9

Library of Congress Control Number: 2007905051

DEDICATION

Irene Jewel Dellon

August 21, 1918 – October 13, 1989

My Mom, an Optometrist, Math Teacher, and Optimist, taught me the love
of learning, and understanding of basic principles that continue enabling me
to create, write and teach. She was also a Type II Diabetic.

Alfred L. Dellon

February 11, 1915 – October 14, 1988

My Dad, an Engineer, Consultant, and Pragmatist, told me to "get your head
out of the book and look around you. Be aware of what is going on in the real
world too," and "Do Not Quit."

Irene and Al Dellon in Luxemborg in 1986. They loved to travel, and are still together.

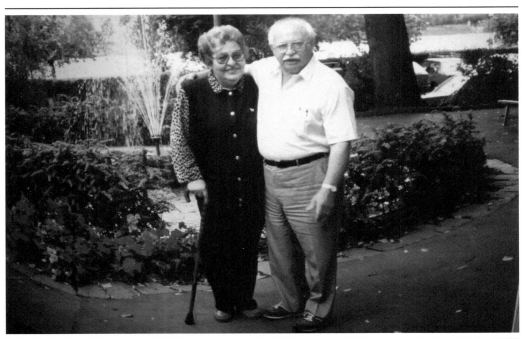

ACKNOWLEDGEMENTS

It is with more than just fatherly pride that I state the obvious: This book owes its artistic design, precision layout and intrinsic coherence, from cover design, to page format and bar graphs, to the creative and meticulous work of Glenn George Dellon. Glenn, thanks so much, and a big hug and kiss. And it is with more than just a husband's love that I state what might not be so obvious: This book owes its very existence to the gift of time from our lives together that Luiann Olivia Greer has given. This creation, *Pain Solutions,* has been born under her watchful and critical eye during our travels together, beginning first at the One and Only Ocean Club on Paradise Island in the Bahamas in December of 2005, and being completed at the Marina Grand Hotel on Mykonos, in Greece in June of 2007. Her gift of time, like her love, is precious. Luiann, thanks, and love you forever.

1

Chapter One
Why Nerves Cause Pain

"It is okay to
lose your nerve."

Pain Solutions

Pain Solutions is a book to help you understand there is hope that your pain can be greatly relieved, and, sometimes, completely eliminated by the appropriate peripheral nerve surgery. Surgery, of course, is the last resort. If you are reading this book, then most likely you have already had all the usual non-surgical treatments for your pain. By describing how individuals, like you, have been helped, I hope to make this book personally important to you or someone you know.

In this chapter, I outline the basic mechanisms of pain related to conditions for which I have developed pain solutions. In the chapters that follow specific solutions are discussed for your pain.

If you have pain, then impulses are traveling along a nerve into your spine. From your spine those impulses continue to your brain. Pain is a message that there is a problem somewhere in your body to which you need to pay attention. You may not like the pain message, but it calls your attention to a problem. *Pain Solutions* will help you find the answers that perhaps your own caring physician(s) have not been able to find for you.

The central nervous system consists of the brain and spinal cord. Problems in the brain are usually related to tumors, bleeding, or lack of blood supply (stroke). These usually cause headache and loss of some function, but they do not usually cause pain in your arms or legs, or your body. Problems in the spinal cord can cause pain in these areas of your body by having some part of the boney or ligamentous spine cause pressure on the spinal cord or nerve roots. It is usually pretty clear that this pain is coming from your neck or back. Traditional x-rays, the newer MRIS (special imaging studies), or traditional electrodiagnostic studies usually can identify this problem. An example of nerve root compression and imaging for the spine in the neck, the cervical spine is given in Figure 3-1. These symptoms can be treated often without surgery, but sometimes portions of the vertebral column must be removed, like a disc, or the bone alongside the nerve (a laminectomy). If the bone is not stable, the spine may have to be fused at some level. These operations are done by Neurosurgeons or Orthopedic

Surgeons. This type of pain usually has a special pattern to it. A well known one for the lower extremity "sciatica," where the pain goes from the back, into the buttocks, and thighs, and can extend all the way to the toes. An example in the upper extremity might be the compression of the nerve root between the 5TH and 6TH cervical vertebra, which causes pain from the neck, into the shoulder, and down towards the index finger. Certain muscles, like the biceps for elbow flexion, might be weak. A reflex might be lost. In this situation, pressure applied to the top of the head down into the neck can cause the symptoms, and this is called a positive Spurling sign (see Figure 1-2). When the pain is caused by problems in the central nervous system, the peripheral nerves are not tender.

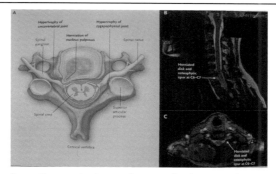

Figure 1-1. Left: Illustration of a cervical vertebra in which examples of the intervertebral disc is compressing the nerve root on the left side and bone is compressing it on the right. The spinal cord is noted in the center. Right: Examples of magnetic resonance imaging (MRI) of the cervical spine showing the problem that exists at (left). (With permission from the New England Journal of Medicine article Cervical Radiculopathy, Volume 353, pages 392-399, 2005, by S. Carette, and M.G., Fehlings.

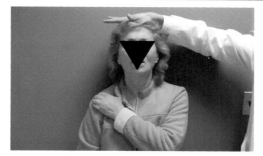

Figure 1-2. A positive Spurling sign occurs when pressure applied to the top of the head results in pain going into the shoulder or fingers, such as illustrated here. This is a sign of cervical nerve root compression.

The Peripheral Nervous System consists of all the nerves that are outside of the brain and the spinal cord: the nerves in your arms and legs, and in your face and in your chest and abdomen. In general, there are three main problems or events that happen to peripheral nerves that cause them to send a pain message to your brain. These three categories are neuroma, nerve compression, and neuropathy. Let us first define what these are and give you some common examples so that you may see that there is hope to stop the pain message by correcting directly the problem with the nerve itself at the point at which the pain message starts. When the pain is coming from the peripheral nerves, there is usually a spot along the path of a nerve that you can touch which causes that pain (see Figure 1-3).

The Peripheral Nerve surgeons of the Dellon Institutes for Peripheral Nerve Surgery® are especially trained to identify these sources of pain. (Visit us at Dellon.com). Let us understand each pain source better.

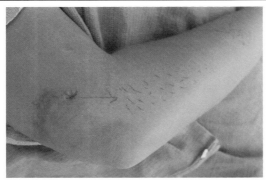

Figure 1-3. The brownish region is where this upper arm and elbow were injured at work. The * on the skin is where pain occurs when that spot is touched. The dotted area is where the pain travels when the painful spot is touched. There is also less feeling in this region. This indicates injury to a peripheral nerve. The painful spot has a neuroma. This patient can be helped by removing the neuroma (see Figure 1-4.).

Neuroma

For the rest of *Pain Solutions,* a peripheral nerve will be called simply a "nerve." A nerve begins in the spinal cord and extends to somewhere in the body, for example the index finger tip. Whenever a nerve is injured, it tries to grow back to where it originally was. This is called nerve regeneration. Peripheral nerves do regenerate. They are wrapped by small cells described by Theodore Schwann (1810-1882), the father of cellular biology. He did not know what they do. In fact they were thought to be part of the nerve cell itself. Today we know that they are totally different cells. They make myelin, which is the insulation covering the individual nerve fibers that permits them to conduct an impulse quickly to the brain from the point at which the nerve is stimulated.

When a nerve is injured, the part farthest away from the spinal cord, the axon, dies, but the Schwann cell still lives. The Schwann cell is not attached to the spinal cord. The actual origin of the nerve fiber in the spinal cord is still alive, and wants to heal the part of the nerve that was injured. When the nerve fiber degenerates, the Schwann cell makes nerve growth factor, which attracts the nerve fiber to grow back across the site of injury and reconnect to where it used to go (see Figure 1-4).

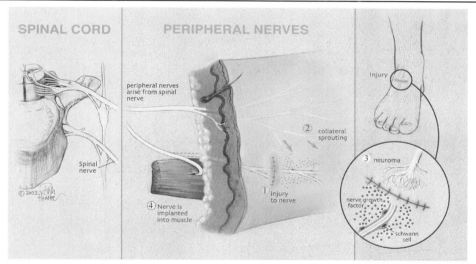

Figure 1-4. Nerve fibers arise in the spinal cord (left panel), leave the vertebral foramen to become peripheral nerves (center panel). When an injury occurs, as in (1), the part of the nerve traveling past the injury site dies. In the right panel, Schwann cells are noted around the nerve fiber, and they begin to produce nerve growth factor to attract or call the nerve to grow back, or regenerate. When the nerve fibers get stuck in the scar while attempting to grow back, they form a neuroma (3). In the center panel, a normal nearby nerve is affected by the nerve growth factor and creates new nerve sprouts which can grow in to the denervated territory, a process called collateral sprouting. In (4) the process of implanting a nerve into muscle is shown. This is the technique used by the Dellon Institutes for Peripheral Nerve Surgery® to prevent a painful neuroma. (With permission from http://www.dellon.com)

The injured nerve can actually grow pretty fast, about one inch per month. When the spinal cord is injured, the nerve fibers within the spinal cord have trouble regenerating because they contain a different form of myelin and they do not have Schwann cells to make nerve growth factor. In fact, there are small cells in the spinal cord that make a substance that prevents nerve regeneration within the spinal cord. This is why a person with a broken neck, as happened falling off a horse to Christopher Reeves (who played the character Superman in the movies), usually remains paralyzed. One day we will know how to reverse this process and permit healing within the spinal cord. Today, however, only the peripheral nerves regenerate.

When a peripheral nerve regenerates back along the same pathway it originally had, sensory and motor function can be restored. It may not be normal sensory and motor function, but useful function can be restored. When a peripheral nerve regenerates into scar, it is blocked. The small nerve fibers become trapped in the fibrous scar tissue and form a painful neuroma. This is illustrated in Figure 1-4.

It is Okay to Lose Your Nerve

"Doctor Dellon," said Carmen, "ever since that door crushed my elbow, I have had pain that shoots into my forearm whenever that spot is touched. It happened at work two years ago. I cannot even let the therapist touch it, because it just hurts too much. Can you help me?"

Carmen's arm is shown in Figure 1-3. The door had cut the skin when it crushed her arm, leaving a thick brown scar where the emergency room doctor had sewn the skin closed. She had an area of skin that felt unusual when touched (the dotted area) and a trigger point that sent the pain downwards towards that unhappy (dysesthetic) skin. This meant Carmen had a neuroma of a nerve to the skin.

"Yes, Carmen, I can fix that. I need to make a new incision along the length of the nerve that is injured, find the neuroma, which is the damaged end of the nerve, and implant that nerve into a muscle to prevent it from growing back again," I explained.

I showed her the illustration in Figure 1-4, which is one prepared especially for the Dellon Institutes for Peripheral Nerve Surgery®.

"Doctor Dellon, I want you to do the surgery," Carmen replied. "How long will it be until I can use my hand again? When will I know I am better?"

"You can use your hand right after surgery. When you wake up from surgery, you will know your pain from the neuroma is gone. There will just be the pain from the surgery itself."

"My pain is gone, Doctor Dellon. I can touch my elbow again. You were right. It was okay to lose my nerve."

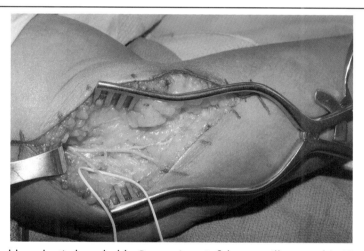

Figure 1-5. The blue plastic loop holds Carmen's painful nerve, illustrated in Figure 1-3.

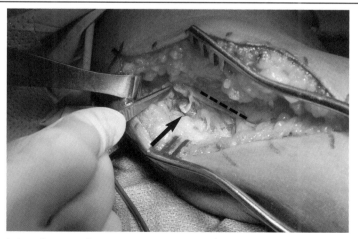

Figure 1-6. The injured nerve shown in Figures 1-3 and 1-6 is buried in muscle (arrow) to prevent it again from causing pain. The rest of the nerve has been preserved (dotted line).

YOU SHOULD HAVE YOUR PAINFUL NERVE REMOVED IF: You have had pain for more than 6 months; The function of the nerve is not critical (if its function is critical, the nerve should be reconstructed); You have not responded to non-operative treatments such as anti-inflammatory drugs, steroid injection, opiates or neuropathic pain medication (gabapentin); You have had relief of pain following a nerve block.

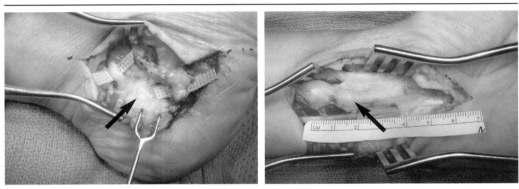

Figure 1-7. Examples of neuromas. The heel, where the calcaneal nerve was injured during surgery for plantar fasciitis (arrow, left), and of the wrist, where median nerve was injured in a suicide attempt (arrow, right).

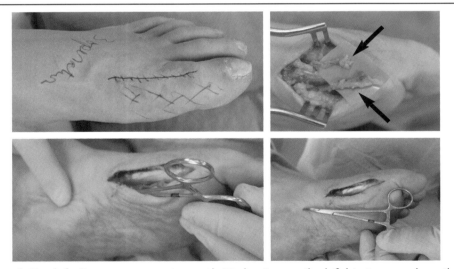

Figure 1-8. Top left: Surgery to correct an arthritic bunion on the left big toe was done three times. The toe is now straight, and the joint deformity corrected, but the striped area near the incision is painful. At surgery (top right) two separate injured nerves are shown, each with a painful neuroma (arrows). The treatment is to remove the painful neuroma, and to take the end of the nerve (bottom left) and implant it into a muscle (bottom right), the location of which is shown by the pointing clamp. The muscle is an area where no pressure occurs while walking.

Nerve Compression

Compression of a nerve is very common. The name of the commonest site of nerve compression is now almost a household word: Carpal Tunnel Syndrome. Almost everyday, you will see someone wearing a splint on their wrist to keep the wrist straight, preventing it from bending over and compressing the median nerve. Almost everyone knows someone who has had carpal tunnel surgery. Decompression of the median nerve at the wrist may be the most common operation done in the United States. About 500,000 of these operations are done almost every year. About 125 out of every 100,000 people in the United States will get carpal tunnel syndrome during their lifetime. The surgery is successful in about 85% of people in relieving their symptoms.

The commonest symptom of carpal tunnel syndrome is that you wake up at night with your thumb, index and middle fingers asleep, but sometimes it seems as if the whole hand is asleep. With time, these three fingers become numb most of the day. In the advanced condition, some of the thumb muscles become weak, and may atrophy.

The initial treatment of chronic nerve compression is NOT surgery. First, daily activity that prolongs wrist flexion is altered. For example, the position in which you hold your wrist while typing on the computer should be altered so it is not so bent. Next, you will take an anti-inflammatory medication to reduce swelling of the tissues that surround the tendons within the carpal tunnel (there are nine such tendons that move the fingers). This tissue can become swollen and stuck to the median nerve with injury or arthritis or over-use. You will wear a splint to keep the wrist from bending, especially at night. You may receive an injection of steroid into the carpal tunnel to shrink the swollen tissues (but do not have the nerve itself injected!).

Finally, surgical decompression of the carpal tunnel will be done (see Figure 1-9). This surgery is done today through a small incision, but is illustrated with a longer incision that permits demonstration of the indentation of the median nerve and the removal of the scar tissue around the nerve (neurolysis).

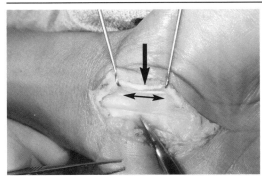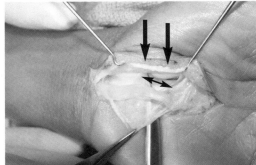

Figure 1-9. Left: The carpal tunnel is opened widely at the wrist in this example of decompression of the median nerve (arrow) at the wrist for treatment of carpal tunnel syndrome. The region of compression can clearly be seen at the end of the clamp (double arrow). The divided edge of the ligament that was causing compression, the transverse carpal ligament is the white edge indicated by the small arrows (Left and Right). This surgery can be done through a much smaller incision. Right: The clamp holds the scarred covering of the median nerve, which is removed during this neurolysis. The narrowed area of the median nerve is still noted (double arrows).

Between a Rock and a Hard Place

A nerve is a soft structure that goes from the spine to either muscle or skin. Along the pathway from its origin to its destination, the nerve passes by ligaments and bones. In many locations, the passageway between the ligament and the bone is narrow. When the nerve passes through such a narrow region, it is between a rock and a hard place. The nerve can become compressed in this area.

Nerve compression means the pressure on the nerve is increased. This causes blood flow in the nerve to decrease. Decreased blood flow in the nerve results in too little oxygen. When the nerve gets too little blood flow, the nerve sends a message to the brain, asking for help. This message makes you feel like your hand is buzzing , or tingling, or "falling asleep."

If you are being choked, your brain does not get oxygen, and you will collapse and become unconscious. When a nerve does not get oxygen, it stops conducting normal electrical impulses. When this occurs , it is like the electricity going off in your house; the lights flicker, and then go out.

When you awaken at night with your "hand asleep," or buzzing, it is because the nerves at the wrist or elbow are compressed, and the lack of oxygen to the nerve sends the message that awakens you.

When you cross your legs, and your top leg "goes to sleep," it is because the nerve on the outside of the knee is getting compressed and sends the message to warn you of this problem. If this problem persists, you have weakness in your foot, and it feels as if you can hardly take a step.

When the pressure on the nerve is sudden and heavy, you experience pain as well as buzzing. But if the pressure comes on slowly, and lasts a long time, and continues for many months, you do not have pain. Just numbness that comes and goes, and then the skin supplied by the nerve stays numb and loses its feeling. This is chronic nerve compression.

The Dellon Institutes for Peripheral Nerve Surgery® specialize in decompression of nerves in both the upper and lower extremities. Descriptions of some of these operations are available to download from our website at Dellon.com. Brochures are available on these subjects:

Carpal Tunnel Syndrome

Cubital Tunnel Syndrome

Radial Nerve Entrapments

Brachial Plexus Compression (Thoracic Outlet Syndrome)

Tarsal Tunnels Syndrome

Foot Drop

Heel Pain Syndromes

The research models I helped to develop in the early 1980's demonstrated that within 2 months of nerve compression, fluid begins to leak from blood vessels into the nerve, that by 6 months of compression, the myelin protein covering the nerve fibers begins to get damaged, and that by one year, nerve fibers have begun to die. Scar tissue forms between the bundles within the large nerve.* The nerve itself, may become stuck to the surrounding ligaments. Once this degree of scar tissue forms, only surgery can relieve pressure on the nerve sufficiently to relieve symptoms.

Surgery must relieve pressure on the compressed nerve. Either the rock or the hard place must be removed, or the nerve itself must be moved to place without a rock or a hard place to compress it.

---

*References to research on nerve compression from the 1980's:

*Dellon AL, Kallman CH: Evaluation of functional sensation in the hand. J Hand Surg 8:865-870, 1983.

*Mackinnon SE, Dellon AL, Hudson AR, Hunter D: Chronic nerve compression – an experimental model in the rat. Ann Plast Surg 13:112-120, 1984.

*Mackinnon SE, Dellon AL, Daneshvar A: Histopathology of the tarsal tunnel syndrome: Examination of a human tibial nerve. Contemp Orthop 9:43-48, 1984.

*Mackinnon SE, Dellon AL, Hudson AR, Hunter DA: A primate model for chronic nerve compression. J Reconstr Microsurg 1:185-194, 1985.

*Mackinnon SE, Dellon AL, Hudson AR, Hunter DA: Histopathology of compression of the superficial radial nerve in the forearm. J Hand Surg 11A:206-209, 1986.

*Dellon AL: Musculotendinous variations about the elbow. J Hand Surg 11B:175-181, 1986.

An example of removing one of the hard places is given for the carpal tunnel in Figure 1-9. An example of moving the nerve to a new place is given for ulnar nerve compression at the elbow, Cubtial Tunnel Syndrome, in Figure 1-10.

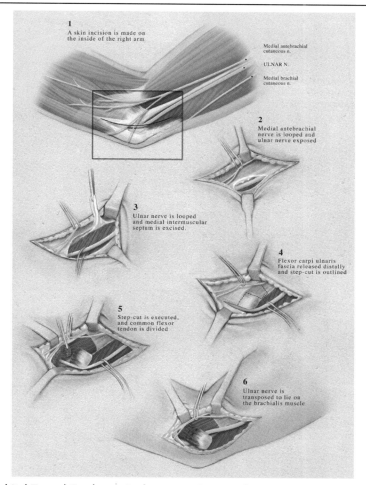

Figure 1-10. Cubital Tunnel Syndrome is the name given to ulnar nerve compression at the elbow. Symptoms of numbness in the little and ring finger, weakness of pinch and grasp, and of clumsiness or dropping objects are corrected by moving the ulnar nerve from between the two bones and ligament that cause the compression. The operation I developed for this purpose is illustrated here. The ulnar nerve is seen moving from its location behind the elbow in (5) to a new place created for it in front of the elbow (6). The muscles are lengthened (4) to provide a large place for the ulnar nerve. Immediate elbow movement is permitted to prevent scar tissue from making the nerve stuck in the new location. The most recent report of success with this operation notes more than 600 patients treated without recurrence of symptoms (Dellon AL, Coert JH: Technique of musculofascial lengthening for treatment of ulnar nerve compression at the elbow. J Bone Joint Surgery, 86A: 169-179, 2004., with permission from http://ww.Dellon.com)

Figures 1-11 and 1-12 show examples of different nerve decompressions.

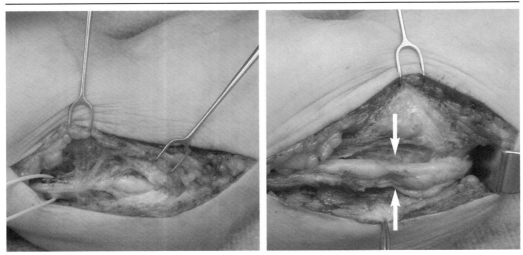

Figure 1-11. Example of ulnar nerve compression at the right elbow. Left: This nerve is entrapped in scar tissue overlying the site where the elbow was bruised in a fall. Right: The site of indentation of the ulnar nerve is noted by the white arrow, with swelling of the nerve in either side of the entrapment. After completion of this neurolysis stage of the surgery, the ulnar nerve will be transposed to lie beneath the lengthened flexor-pronator muscle mass using Dr. Dellon's operation (Figure 1-10).

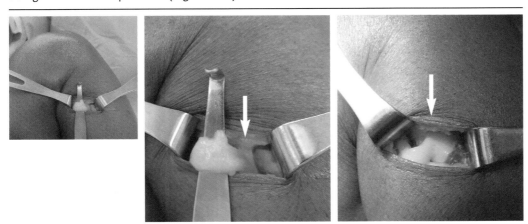

Figure 1-12. Example of nerve compression of the common peroneal nerve at the knee. Left: overall view to orient the surgical view. The incision is located at the boney prominence of the fibular, where the site of compression is. This patient injured the outside of this knee. Center: The metal retractor is underneath the large nerve, which is white in color in contrast the appearance (yellow) noted in patients with diabetes or some forms of neuropathy. The band that is compressing the nerve is noted by the white arrow. Right: the compressive band has been removed. The white arrow points to the indentation or notch in the common peroneal nerve at the site of compression by the band. With pressure gone from the nerve, sensation and strength will return to the leg and foot.

Documentation of Nerve Compression

"Doctor Dellon," my medical doctor sent me to a neurologist to see if my symptoms of numbness were due to a nerve compression. The neurologist said I had to have nerve conduction testing and electromyography. The NCV and EMG really hurt! The test cost about $1,600. And after all that the Neurologist said I was 'normal! But I really have a problem Doctor Dellon. Isn't there some test that can identify my nerve problem?

This patient's experience is all too common. The traditional electrodiagnostic testing was developed in the 1950's. It gives electrical stimulus, or shocks to the nerves through the skin, and sometimes actual needles are inserted into the skin and the response to the shock is recorded through the needle. Of course this hurts, and is very expensive. Unfortunately, because this test measures the speed of electrical activity in the fastest nerve fibers, a lot of nerve fibers can be injured or not working and the test still shows a normal measurement. This electrical test is simply not sensitive enough to identify many nerve compressions. The electromyography is still necessary if your doctor is evaluating a nerve root compression in your neck or a primary muscle disease. An MRI, a special form of x-ray will be necessary to image your spinal cord.

This is a subject I have written extensively about for many years. My most recent writing on this subject compares traditional electrodiagnostic testing to a test that I developed in 1989 and have been proving the value of ever since.* This neurosensory test is non-painful, has no needles, and is not expensive. The testing instrument is called the Pressure-Specified Sensory Device™ (PSSD). Here is how it works.

You are seated comfortably in a chair, and the PSSD is touched to your finger tip, your toe, or your lip (see Figure 11-4). The two rounded metal prongs are pressed gently into the skin. You press a button when you can feel the pressure for the first time and when you can tell whether one or two tips are pressing the skin. This does not hurt. By comparing how hard you had

---

*Dellon AL: Measuring Peripheral Nerve Function: Neurosensory Testing versus Electrodiagnostic Testing, in Atlas of the Hand Clinics: Nerve Repair and Reconstruction, D. Slutsky, editor, Elsevier, Philadelphia, Chapter 1, pp 1-31, 2005.

to be touched to feel the prongs, and how close together you could tell you were being touched, the PSSD results give us the information to know whether you have nerve compression and whether the nerve is dying (see Figure 1-16.) If the nerve has begun to die, which means you cannot tell when two points are touching the skin close together, then it is time for surgery to decompress the nerves.

Neuropathy

"Neuropathy" is best understood to be a problem with the nerves in your body, in contrast to a neuroma or a nerve compression, which is a problem with a single nerve in your body. If your median nerve is injured, you can have a neuroma of the median nerve, somewhere along its path, on either your left or your right side (see Figure 1-7 right). If you have a compression of your median nerve, you have an area at which this nerve is compressed, for example at your wrist (carpal tunnel syndrome, see Figure 1-9). About 50% of people have carpal tunnel syndrome bilaterally, which is on both sides of your body, your right and your left hand. The carpal tunnel syndrome on the right side may be worse than your left side. If all the fingers of both your right and left hands are equally numb and/or painful, then you have a neuropathy. Something systemic in your body is affecting your peripheral nerves. You have a peripheral neuropathy.

The most common cause of a peripheral neuropathy is diabetes. Other common causes of neuropathy are thyroid disorders: if the thyroid function is low, then water accumulates in your nerves, making them swell and causing them to become compressed in regions with tight anatomic tunnels like the wrist and ankle. Another cause of neuropathy are diseases in which the body attacks itself with antibodies, like lupus and rheumatoid arthritis; the inflammation along the blood vessels (vasculitis) in the nerves makes them susceptible to compression at known sites of anatomic narrowing like the wrist and ankle. Another cause of neuropathy is poisoning by heavy metals, like arsenic, lead, and mercury: these cause fluid to leak from the blood vessels into the inside of the nerve, making it susceptible to compression at known sites of anatomic narrowing like the wrist and ankle.

Chemotherapy drugs used to fight cancer, like, vincristine, taxol, cisplatin, and thalidomide, can slow down the transport of critical molecules within the nerve. Again, this makes the nerve susceptible to compression. It is clear that neuropathy, what ever its cause, may create symptoms through mechanisms similar to those that give symptoms with a single nerve compression, and this gives us a cause for optimism, a cause for hope. In many people with neuropathy, there are compressed nerves that are responsible for most of the symptoms. If this is true, then these symptoms, attributed to neuropathy, can be relieved by decompression of nerves.

Stocking and Glove

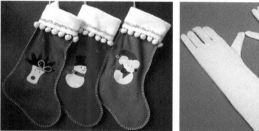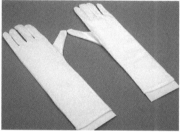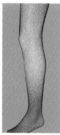

Figure 1-13. A peripheral neuropathy causes loss of sensation and or pain in a specific pattern. In the legs the pattern is that of a stocking. In the arms it is the pattern of a glove. A stocking pattern can be created by compression of several nerves in the leg and ankle, and a glove pattern can be created by compression of several nerves in the arm and wrist. Compressed nerves can be decompressed, creating the possibility of hope for neuropathy.

Usually, with a peripheral neuropathy, your feet become involved, symptomatic, first. The feet are involved in both the top and bottom of your feet, and the symptoms extend up the ankle, in what is the pattern of a stocking. When the neuropathy is in the upper extremities, it occurs in the pattern you would have if you were wearing gloves.

In the upper extremity, if you combine compression of the ulnar nerve at the elbow (cubital tunnel syndrome), compression of the radial nerve in the forearm (radial sensory nerve compression), and compression of the median nerve at the wrist (cubital tunnel syndrome) you will have a pattern of sensory loss that fits a glove. As you now know, from reading above, a compressed nerve can be decompressed by surgery, relieving pain and numbness in most patients. The same thinking applies to the leg and foot.

In the lower extremity, if you combine compression of the common peroneal nerve at the knee (fibular tunnel syndrome), compression of the deep peroneal nerve over the top of the foot (described by me in 1990), and compression of the tibial nerves and its branches in the four medial (inside of) ankle tunnels (tarsal tunnels syndrome), you will have a pattern of sensory loss that fits like a stocking. As you now know, compressed nerves can be decompressed with surgery, relieving pain and numbness in most patients. This is discussed in detail in Chapter 2.

New "Ropathy"

"I have neuropathy?," the patient with diabetes asked her doctor. "I have numbness and burning in my hands and feet. Is it going to get better? Can you help me?"

" I am sorry Mrs. Brown," her doctor answered, "Certainly I can help you keep your blood sugar under control, and I can give you medicine for the pain, but neuropathy is progressive and irreversible" he informed her.

"PROGRESSIVE AND IRREVERSIBLE." For decades, this was the correct answer in medical school, the correct answer on a medical exam, and the answer given to patients. "Neuropathy is progressive and irreversible" means there is no hope. If your medical problem is hopeless, depression and disability is likely.

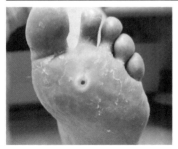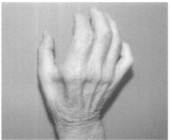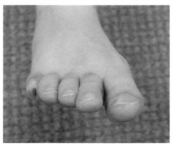

Figure 1-14. Examples of progressive neuropathy. Ulcer beneath the bottom of the second toe (left) and at tip of fifth toe (right) develop because of lack of sensation. Muscle wasting in the hand is noted in the center. The fingers begin to form a "claw" and this can happen in the foot as well. On the right, the toes are beginning to curl up.

"Progressive and irreversible" is the old view of neuropathy.

"Doctor Dellon, I have neuropathy. Can you help me?" This is the e-mail question that comes through my website, Dellon.com so often each day, and through my phone line 1 877-DELLON-1. "Yes, I can help you. In most people who have a nerve compression associated with their neuropathy, the nerve can be decompressed. Symptoms can be relieved in 80% of people."

"Doctor Dellon, will I still be at risk for getting an ulcer or having an amputation," the questions go on.

"If sensation is restored to your feet, you will not have an ulcer, you will NOT have an amputation, and even your balance can be improved," I answer. That is the new neuropathy, or "new-ropathy" as I like to call it.

New-Ropathy is the first good news about neuropathy. It is optimistic. There is hope. "Restore sensation. Relieve Pain."

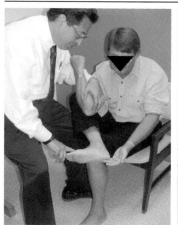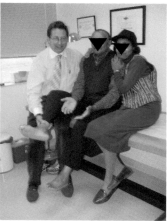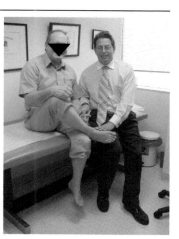

Figure 1-15. Adam, Bob, and Clark, shown above, have had each arm and each leg operated upon to decompress nerves. Every three months for one year, they each had an operation till all four extremities was decompressed. Each has neuropathy still. But each no longer has pain, and each has recovered sensation. They each now have... "New-Ropathy," a systemic disease without the symptoms of nerve compression.

Neurosensory Testing and the PSSD

"Doctor Dellon," the man sitting in my office said, "I know I have neuropathy. I have been to so many doctors. They have done electrical testing that show I have neuropathy, but they say nothing can be done. How did you decide that I have a nerve compression and that I can be helped? How did you decide that I would most likely be better in about three months?"

My new approach to neuropathy, or new-ropathy, is based upon:

The concept that the symptoms of neuropathy can be due to the presence of nerve compression;

The ability to measure peripheral nerve function with the Pressure-Specified Sensory Device™;

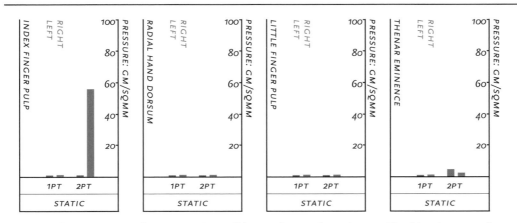

Figure 1-16. PSSD report demonstrating mild carpal tunnel syndrome. The blue bars are for the left side and the red bars are for the right side. Normal bar height is below the black lines, representing low pressure. The far left graph is the index finger, the left-center is the back of the hand, the right-center is the little finger, and the far right is the palm. The right index finger bar is elevated indicating abnormal pressure on the right median nerve. Since there is no * (asterisk) next to the bar, no nerve fibers are dying. This test is consistent with mild right carpal tunnel syndrome. Splinting is advised, not surgery.

Identification of the site of nerve compression along the length of the nerve by knowing where the anatomy can create the tight area, and the ability to determine if the nerve can still regenerate by tapping on the nerve (the presence of a positive Tinel sign);

If there is a tingling into the skin when the nerve is tapped at the site of compression, and the PSSD shows a moderate degree of degeneration, there is an 80% chance of recovery and this recovery usually occurs by three months after surgery. If the PSSD shows more advanced degeneration, then recovery can take up to one year for the nerves to regenerate into the toes.

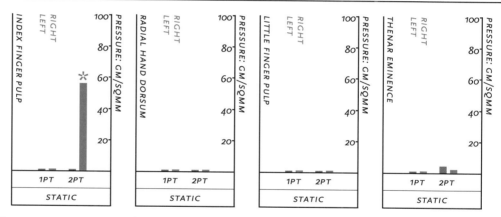

Figure 1-17. PSSD report demonstrating severe carpal tunnel syndrome. The blue bars are for the left side and the red bars are for the right side. Normal bar height is below the black lines, representing low pressure. The far left is the index finger, the left-center is the back of the hand, the right-center is the little finger, and the far right is the palm. The right index finger bar is elevated indicating abnormal pressure on the right median nerve, and there is an * (asterisk) next to the bar; nerve fibers are dying. This test is consistent with severe right carpal tunnel syndrome. Nerve decompression is advised.

Figure 1-16 and 1-17 should be compared to Figure 1-18 below to see the difference in appearance of the results of testing with the PSSD. It is clear that chronic nerve compression can easily be differentiated from a neuropathy, and the degree of these nerve problems can be determined as well. This painless testing with the PSSD documents your peripheral nerve problem and helps your doctor plan your treatment.

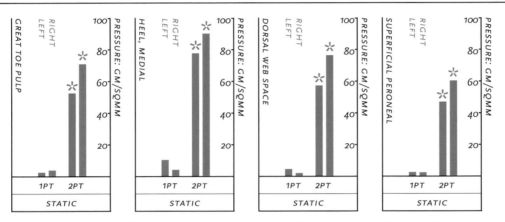

Figure 1-18. PSSD report demonstrating neuropathy. The blue bars are for the left side and the red bars are for the right side. Normal bar height is below the black lines, representing low pressure. The four skin territories tested represent the big toe (far left) and the heel (left-center), innervated by the tibial nerve, in the tarsal tunnel, and the two areas on the top of the foot (right-center and far right), innervated by the peroneal nerve. Note that the bars are elevated for the left and the right side of the top and the bottom of the foot, indicating a problem with multiple nerves, to the same degree on each side of the body. This is the pattern of a neuropathy, such as that seen in diabetes. The elevated bars are for two-point static touch, the first test to become abnormal with nerve compression or neuropathy. Other traditional testing would still indicate the nerves are normal. The small plastic filaments, called Semmes-Weinstein nylon monofilaments, attempt to give a measure of one point static touch, which is similar to the low bars on the left of each graph. Note that this measurement is still normal, so that the nylon filament test would still say this patient had normal sensation even though the PSSD demonstrates neuropathy. The asterisks indicate that nerve fibers are dying at each site tested. This result demonstrates a sensory neuropathy with axonal loss, but is also consistent with nerve entrapments at the knee, the top of the foot, and the ankle region. Decompression of these nerves offers hope for relief of the symptoms attributed to neuropathy.

Pain Solutions Summary

There are three categories of problems that can occur with a peripheral nerve, and each can be helped by approaches I have developed. The three categories of nerve problems are:

1. Neuroma which is an actual injury to the nerve.

2. Nerve Compression which is localized area of pressure.

3. Neuropathy which is systemic disease that affects the nerves in the body, usually the legs and feet worse, then the hands, but which also can make the nerves more likely to become compressed at predictable locations.

My research into peripheral nerve problems over the past 25 years has demonstrated that:

Painful neuromas can be removed. Scarring can be removed from compressed nerves.

Even in the presence of neuropathy, areas of tightness, *causing chronic nerve compression,* can be opened about the nerves, restoring sensation, relieving pain, preventing ulceration and amputation, and permitting balance to recover. This is the new news about neuropathy.

Go to Dellon.com or call +1 877-DELLON-1 (+1 877-335-5661) for more information.

2

Chapter Two
Neuropathy
Related to Diabetes

"There is horrible burning pain and numbness in my feet. Medicines are not helping me. I don't want an ulcer or an amputation."

The News

"Read all about it!, Read all about it! The latest news about Neuropathy!," shouts the newspaper boy standing on the street corner. And the millions of people throughout the world with neuropathy stop and take a copy of the paper. There is no charge for this SPECIAL EDITION OF THE NEWS. It is given out as a public service announcement world wide:

"A. Lee Dellon, MD wrote in 1988* that there was a new "OPTIMISM" for those with neuropathy. The underlying medical problem, like DIABETES, makes the nerves in the arms and legs more likely to get compressed in the natural tunnels at the wrist and elbow, ankle and knee. Compressed nerves gives symptoms of numbness, weakness, and pain. Dr. Dellon developed operations to remove the pressure from these nerves NOW.

PAIN CAN BE RELIEVED! SENSATION RESTORED! ULCERS CAN BE PREVENTED! AMPUTATION CAN BE PREVENTED! BALANCE REGAINED! TODAY WE SHOULD THINK OF A 'NEW-ROPATHY.'

"Doctor Dellon," said Rosita, a 48 year old Hispanic woman from California, "why doesn't everyone know yet that people like me can be helped?" She was consulting me in the Dellon Institute located in San Francisco.

"How have you been helped, Rosita," I asked her.

"Doctor Dellon, just three months ago you operated on my right foot. When I came to see you I had horrible pain in both my feet, like I was walking on broken glass," she paused, remembering her difficulty in describing her problem, "and yet, Dr. Dellon, it was so strange because my feet were without much feeling, almost like I was walking on a sponge or blocks of wood. My feet have been like that for two years. That is when my medical doctor told me for the first time that I had diabetes and that I had neuropathy," replied Rosita.

"What did your medical doctor do to help you then Rosita?"

"Doctor Dellon, he made me so scarred! He told me all I could do was get my blood sugar under control with medication and diet, lose weight, and

---

*Dellon AL: Optimism in diabetic neuropathy. Ann Plast Surg 20:103-105, 1988.

he gave me medication usually used for depression and seizures to control my pain," she paused again, remembering her frustration, "But Doctor Dellon, those medications made my head spin. Already I have lost my balance and I fallen." She paused yet again, afraid to tell me the worst news, "Doctor Dellon, she said that I now have one out of six chances to get an ulcer, and then an amputation. I am supposed to look at my feet with a mirror. What I have, the medical doctor said, Neuropathy, is progressive and irreversible. There is no hope for me."

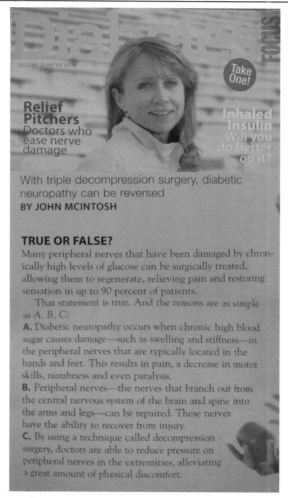

Figure 2-1. News from Diabetes Focus issue second quarter 2006. Article features a Plastic Surgeon from New Jersey, trained by Dr Dellon to do this Triple Nerve Decompression surgery to relieve the symptoms of nerve compression in patients with diabetic neuropathy. The News about the "New-Ropathy" is finally getting out!

"Rosita, I understand why your medical Doctor got you so scared," I said. When I examined you, I found that you had nerve compressions at your knee, the top of your foot, and your ankle. "Now that you have had my operation, which, as you know, we call the "THE DELLON TRIPLE NERVE DECOMPRESSION," how does your right leg feel, the one I operated on, compared to your left leg?"

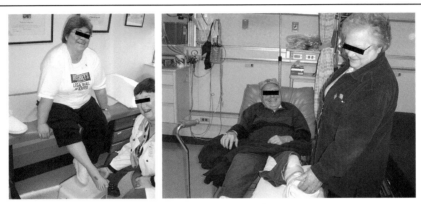

Figure 2-2. Two patients having their operated foot tickled. On the left, two weeks after having the Dellon Triple Nerve Decompression Procedure. On the right, in the recovery room. About half of the people who have this surgery appreciate increased sensation and relief of pain in the early post-surgery time period. Balance is restored when sensation returns. With return of sensation, the neuropathy progression stops. There are no ulcers or amputations.

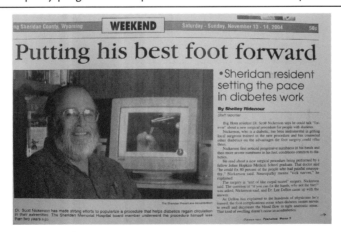

Figure 2-3. Doctor Scott Nickerson, an Orthopedic Surgeon, himself a diabetic, had the Dellon Triple Nerve Decompression procedure on both of his feet by Dr. Dellon. Dr. Nickerson has been greatly improved and now lectures to get the "News," the Optimism about neuropathy, out to the public in his own state of Wyoming, and to the diabetic community at large. A foot being tested painlessly with the Pressure-Specified Sensory Device™ (PSSD), is shown on his computer screen in the background.

"Doctor Dellon, now at 3 months since your surgery, the pain is almost gone in my right foot, and I can feel it when you touch the bottom of my right foot. My left leg, without surgery, still feels the same. Doctor Dellon, how soon can you do the surgery on my other foot? Then I can stop taking all these pain medications. Doctor Dellon, you have given me hope."

And from across the USA, the "News" is making headlines.

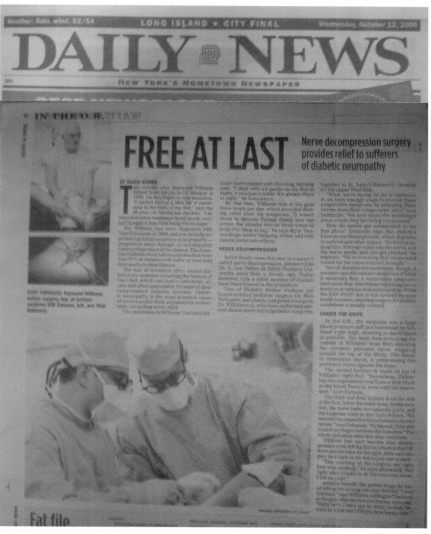

Figure 2-4. Two surgeons in New York City, trained by Dr. Dellon were in the News for their work with the Dellon Triple Nerve Decompression surgery. The "News" continues to be told that this surgery can relieve pain and restore sensation for patients with neuropathy who also have nerve compression(s) in their legs. This surgery is not for everyone with neuropathy, but for that subgroup that also has nerve compressions.

The Old Neuropathy

If you are reading this you most likely have a form of neuropathy.

There are many kinds, but the most common in the world is due to diabetes. Diabetes costs the health care system in the United States one out of every seven dollars. A large part of this cost goes to paying for pain medication for neuropathy, paying for the cost of healing an ulcer (about $28,000), paying for an amputation (about $40,000), paying for hospitalization for a foot infection (about $100,000), or paying for the cost of a broken hip or wrist (due to a fall from loss of balance).

Half of people with diabetes will get neuropathy after having diabetes for about ten years. Ten percent of people first learn they have diabetes when they see their doctor because of their foot pain. One of six diabetics with neuropathy will develop and ulcer. One of six of these people will have an amputation. Half of those with an amputation on one side will get an amputation on the other side, and then half of these people will be dead in three years.

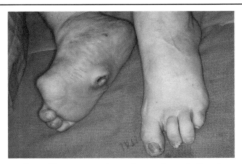

Figure 2-5. The expected results of neuropathy: ulceration, infection, amputation.

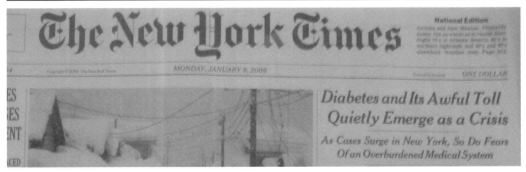

Figure 2-6. Recent News article describing impact of cost of treatment of the complications of Diabetic Neuropathy in the United States. These costs can be reduced greatly by the Dellon Triple Nerve Decompression surgical procedure.

The "Old" Versus "New" Neuropathy Approach

OLD VERSION: NEUROPATHY IS PROGRESSIVE AND IRREVERSIBLE.

With the *old* or traditional approach to neuropathy, the concept was for the medical doctor to treat any underlying known medical cause for the basic disease, like diabetes, and, then to give the patient medication for pain, if pain were part of the neuropathy. As the sensibility became lost, all that could be done was instruction in care for the insensitive foot (using a mirror to look at the bottom of your feet everyday) and wearing special, protective shoes. The neuropathy could be predicted to progress, meaning to get worse, leading to ulceration, infection, amputation, and falls due to loss of balance. In the traditional approach, the doctor did NOT examine the patient for the presence of nerve compressions in the leg or foot. These are NOT present in all patients with neuropathy. Those with and without nerve compressions were thought to be the same and have the same cause for their symptoms.

With the *new* or *Dellon Institute approach to neuropathy,* the concept is that the underlying medical problem makes the peripheral nerves susceptible to compression. This compression may be the primary source of the symptoms. Even if we do not know the cause of the neuropathy,* there is hope for relief of symptoms, because a compressed nerve can be approached with surgery. The site at which the nerve is compressed, or pinched, can be opened.

---

*Idiopathic neuropathy means an unknown cause for the neuropathy.

Decompressing the nerve can relieve symptoms, relieving pain, and restoring sensation. If there is recovery of sensation in the foot, there will not be an ulceration, an infection, or an amputation. **See Figure 2-7 and 2-8 for proof of this statement.**

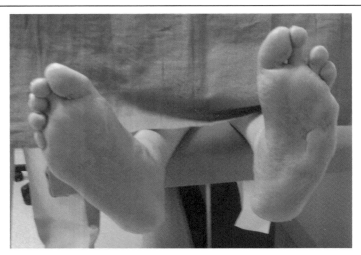

Figure 2-7. Proof that nerve decompression can prevent ulceration and amputation. The right foot had the Dellon Triple Nerve Decompression 15 years ago. The left foot did not have the Dellon approach. The left foot has had the traditional expected result; progressive neuropathy with ulceration and amputation, in this patient, of the fifth toe. In contrast, the right side has maintained sufficient sensation that there has not been ulceration or loss of tissue.

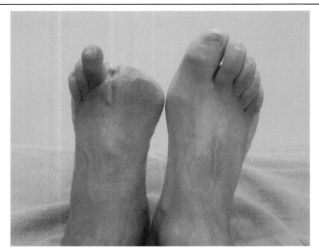

Figure 2-8. Proof that nerve decompression can prevent ulceration and amputation: Right foot had a Dellon Triple Nerve Decompression 7 years ago. Sensation recovered preventing ulceration and amputation. Left foot, without the Dellon Triple Nerve Decompression has developed ulcers, bone infection, and required 2 toe amputations.

Neuropathy can also cause motor weakness and paralysis.

In the "New-Ropathy," the Dellon approach, nerve decompression surgery can also restore muscle function if the muscle has not completely atrophied (died). One of the first muscle functions to be lost, related to the common peroneal nerve next to the knee, is lifting up the big toe (Figure 2-9), and then in time a "foot drop" develops. When this occurs, you may feel like you are stubbing your toe a lot, or dragging your foot, or feel as if your leg is going to give out. In some patients, for reasons that are not understood, once this muscle imbalance occurs, the leg may seem "restless." Once the muscle no longer has a nerve input to it, the muscle begins to atrophy, and then decompression of the nerve may no longer be effective.

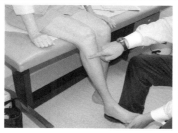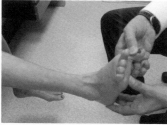

Figure 2-9. Left: Dr. Dellon's finger points to the site of nerve compression near the knee. This is the common peroneal nerve. This nerve provides sensation to the top of the foot and motor function that permits the toes and ankle to lift up. Note area of indentation of the muscle near the finger related to muscle wasting. Right: Dr. Dellon demonstrates weakness in the long toe extensor, the first muscle to become weak with nerve compression. Decompression of the common peroneal nerve at the knee can reverse this weakness and restore strength if the muscle has not become atrophied.

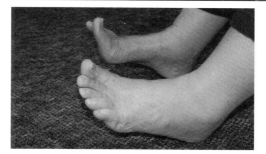

Figure 2-10. The left foot has NOT had surgery. The left big toe is partly paralyzed and does not lift up (extend) completely. Both feet had the same degree of motor weakness and paralysis. The right leg in this photo is three months after a Dellon Triple Nerve Decompression surgery. Note the right big toe can completely extend now after surgery.

When the small muscles in the foot become weak or paralyzed, a "claw foot" develops, as in Figure 2-11 and 2-12. If motor function improves after the nerve decompression surgery, then the paralysis can sometimes be reversed. Figure 2-10 and 2-12 are proof of this statement:

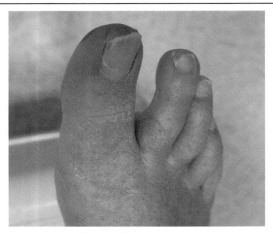

Figure 2-11. The foot of a man with advanced diabetes demonstrates clawing of all toes except the big toe. These toes are hyperextended (bent back towards the foot) because the small muscles that bend the toes are weak or paralyzed. Note skin dryness due to sympathetic (sweating) nerve failure too.

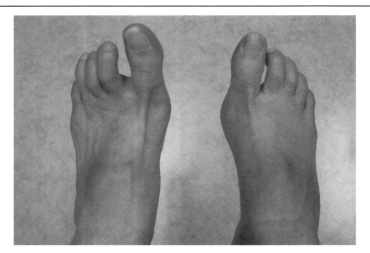

Figure 2-12. Claw & Reversal. The left foot has NOT had surgery. Note that all toes except the big toe are curved back towards the foot, while the tips bend forward, creating a "claw foot" deformity. Six months ago, both feet looked exactly the same. The right foot had a Dellon Triple Nerve Decompression 6 months ago. As strength comes back into the small muscles on the bottom of the foot, innervated by the tibial nerve in the tarsal tunnel, the small toes can regain the strength to flex, removing the claw deformity from the foot.

Restore the Balance to Your Life

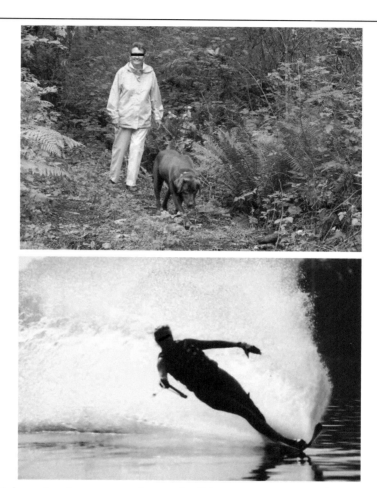

Figure 2-13. Balance has been restored to each of these two patients with neuropathy. Top: This 72 year old woman was no longer able to enjoy even just simply walking her dog in the woods behind her house. Here she is shown doing exactly that after having a Dellon Triple Nerve Decomrpession Surgery on each foot. Bottom: A 27 year old Type I diabetic with severe neuropathy, has regained her balance sufficiently after her Dellon Triple in each leg so that she can resume her favorite activity, water skiing, again.

Get Yourself "New Balance"

Historically, when you lost sensation in your feet, you would lose balance causing falls (Figure 2-9), and perhaps a broken wrist or hip. With the Dellon approach, if you can get your sensation back, your balance can return too. This is demonstrated by the following illustrations in Figures 2-14A and 2-14B.

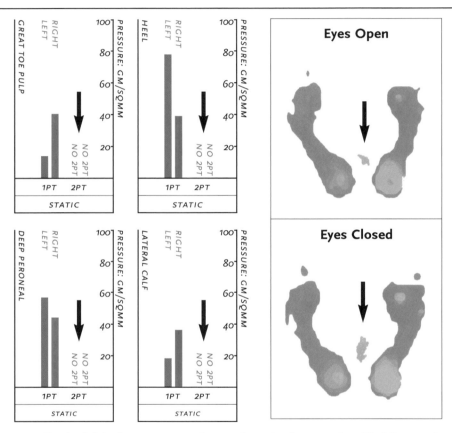

Figure 2-14A. On the left is the computer print out from the Pressure-Specified Sensory Device™ (PSSD) which has documented absence of ability to distinguish one from two touch points (arrows) at four areas of the foot, with the same severe loss of nerves being present both on the left (blue bars) and the right (red bars), which is the picture of an advanced neuropathy. Without sensation, the brain cannot tell in what position to hold the body. On the right, the foot prints obtained from a computer on which the patient is standing, shows the grey area of the center of gravity and how it changes position over 30 seconds. In the top on the right, the patient's eyes are open, and vision is used to maintain the balance. In the bottom on the right, with the eyes closed, the brain must depend on sensory input from the feet, which, as is shown on the left is very poor. Accordingly, the grey outline of the center of gravity increases. This change in center of gravity area is called "sway" and is a measure of loss of balance. This patient, without much sensation due to advanced neuropathy, has increased sway, or decreased balance.

The patient in Figure 2-14A has loss of balance due to loss of sensation. This person cannot stand at night without touching the wall of the bedroom, unless the lights are on. The feet cannot send enough sensory information to the brain. This person falls regularly.

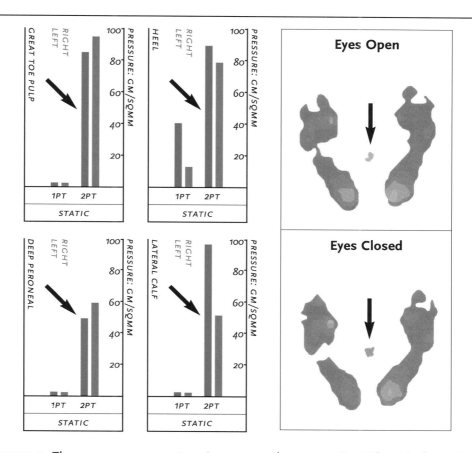

Figure 2-14B. The same measurements as in 2-14A, on the same patient. The right foot is 6 months after a Dellon Triple Nerve Decompression, and the left leg is three months after the same operation. On the left side of the figure, note that the blue and red bars (arrows) on the graph that were absent in Figure 2-14A are now present. This demonstrates that sensation has recovered in the top and bottom of both feet. While the sensation is not yet normal, sensation is greatly improved from before surgery. On the right side of Figure 2-14B, note that the grey area representing the center of gravity, is now about the same with the eyes open and with the eyes closed. Sway is the same with the eyes open or with the eyes closed which is very different than before surgery. Balance is now restored. This means that enough information comes to the brain through the feet that balance is maintained. This patient will no longer fall. In addition to demonstrating that the Dellon Triple Nerve Decompression surgery restores balance, Figures 2-14A and B demonstrate how the Pressure-Specified Sensory Device™ can document the present and stage of neuropathy and also document nerve regeneration during recovery from the surgery.

The Insight

"Doctor Dellon, you have helped my hands, can you help my feet?"

As a Plastic Surgeon who was also a Hand Surgeon, I often would operate on the hands of patients who had nerve problems due to diabetes. About one out of 5 diabetics will develop numbness in the thumb, index and middle finger, that awakens them from sleep. This is called *carpal tunnel syndrome*. These symptoms are due to compression of a nerve the size of a pencil in a tight tunnel in the front of the wrist. The pressure on the nerve causes blood flow to slow down, and when the nerve does not get enough oxygen, the nerve responds by sending a message of numbness or tingling to the brain. Although the existence of this carpal tunnel problem was known in the late 1800's, the first operation to relieve this pressure was probably not done until about 1940, and the surgical release of the ligament across the carpal tunnel to treat carpal tunnel syndrome was not widely accept until the 1950's. Carpal tunnel decompression surgery should give relief of symptoms in 90% of patients. I would do this surgery for my diabetic patients with carpal tunnel syndrome, and they would ask me,

"Doctor Dellon, you have helped my hands, can you help my feet?"

"What is wrong with your feet?" I would answer, because our Plastic Surgery and Hand Surgery training did not teach us much about foot

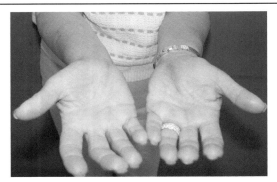

Figure 2-15. "Doctor Dellon, you helped my hands, can you help my feet?" The scars can be seen in the palm of the hands of this woman with neuropathy in her feet and also had carpal tunnel syndrome in each hand. The right hand had decompression of one nerve, the median nerve in the carpal tunnel 6 months before, and left hand had the same surgery 2 months before this photo was taken. The numbness and tingling in her hands are gone. They do not bother her at night. She wanted me to do a nerve decompression on her feet, to give them relief too. Is there a carpal tunnel in the foot?

problems in patients with diabetes. I knew neuropathy existed and led to ulcers, infections and amputations. I knew in neuropathy, sensation was lost in the pattern of glove in the hands and arms, and in the pattern of a stocking in the legs and feet. The problems in the feet usually began first. But the symptoms of carpal tunnel syndrome were in the pattern of just one nerve, the median nerve, while the neuropathy was not the pattern of one nerve.

"Doctor Dellon, my toes feel like my fingers did, but my toes are more numb, and they hurt. The numbness and pain began in my feet and is moving up my leg. Can you help me?" my hand surgery patients would ask?

There were patients with diabetes who had numbness in their little and ring fingers, and clumsiness in their hands. They dropped things. Their hands become weak. The back of their little and ring fingers became numb also. They had ulnar nerve compression at the elbow. This is called *cubital tunnel syndrome*. This problem was known in the late 1800's, but successful surgery to help this problem was not done till about the 1940's, similar to the story of carpal tunnel syndrome. So, I would decompress the ulnar nerve at the elbow, and the patients would say,

"Doctor Dellon, you helped my hands, can you help my feet?"

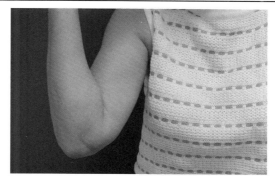

Figure 2-16. The scar at the inside of the elbow is the location for my operation to decompress the ulnar nerve at the elbow in the cubital tunnel. Symptoms from this site of location are numbness in the little and ring finger and part of the back of the hand, and weakness and clumsiness using the hand. This woman, who has neuropathy in her feet, also had cubital tunnel syndrome. Here she is 3 months after ulnar nerve decompression and her symptoms are gone. She wants me to operate to relieve the symptoms in her feet. Is there a cubital tunnel in the leg?

There were patients with diabetes who had numbness and burning over the back of their thumb, index finger and back of their hand. In 1932 there was a report of a diabetic who had these symptoms, but it was thought to be an inflammation of the nerve. In 1986, a site of nerve compression was described by myself and a co-worker.* This site of compression was in the forearm. The compressed nerve is the radial sensory nerve. When this nerve was decompressed, the numbness and burning would go away. "Doctor Dellon, you helped the burning over the back of my forearm and hand, can you help the pain from my knee to the the top of my foot?," asked a diabetic with neuropathy one day after I had helped her arm.

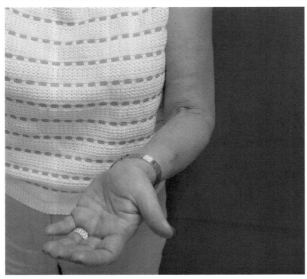

Figure 2-17. Note the small scar just above the bracelet on the left forearm. This is the site of compression of the radial sensory nerve. This woman now has relief of numbness and pain in the back of her forearm, wrist and hand. She had diabetic neuropathy. She wants me to do a similar operation on her leg to help the burning from the knee to the top of the foot. Is there a similar nerve compression in the leg that would make the top of the foot and ankle numb and burn?

*Dellon AL, Mackinnon SE: Radial sensory nerve entrapment in the forearm. J Hand Surg 11A:199-205, 1986.

"Doctor Dellon, you helped my hands, can you help my feet?" This question used to haunt me. Maybe the same type of nerve compressions did occur in the feet, and if they did, maybe the symptoms in the feet of people with neuropathy could be helped by decompressing these nerves. I began to work on identifying an approach to help these feet symptoms:

In the hand, I could decompress three nerves, a *Triple Nerve Decompression,* to give relief in the pattern of a glove. In the leg, could a Triple Nerve Decompression give relief in the pattern of a stocking?

Three nerves sites of compression can give the pattern of a stocking.

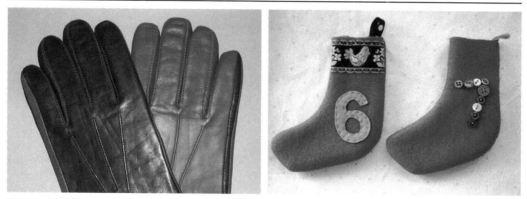

Figure 2-18. If you combine the patterns of the skin affected by compression of the three nerves in the hand and arm, the median nerve in the carpal tunnel, the ulnar nerve in the cubital tunnel, and the radial sensory nerve in the forearm, you get the total sensory area of a glove. What nerve skin patterns would be necessary to give you a stocking? The nerve near the knee, the common peroneal nerve, and tibial nerve, on the inside of the ankle, would give you that pattern. The common peroneal nerve has an entrapment site for one of its branches also in the lower leg and the also on the top of the foot. The tibial nerve has a known description for compression in the tarsal tunnel. Would the same approach I had taken in the hand work in the foot? This was what I had to find out!

The Dellon Triple Nerve Decompression

In 1980, the first patient with a tarsal tunnel syndrome was referred to me. It was first thought by his doctors that his numbness and burning in his feet was due to a circulation problem. Jacob was 73 years old.

"Doctor Dellon," Jacob informed me, "I have retired from many years of public service in our government, and have lived an active life. My health has been great. As I have gotten older, I remember my parents needing to put a blanket around their legs as they got older. They would tell me their feet felt cold, and bothered them at night. They had problems with their balance too. Unfortunately, this has been happening to me for several years now. I thought that maybe modern medicine has found relief for this problem. But the vascular surgeons told me my circulation was great for someone my age, and that maybe you could find a nerve compression in my feet that is giving me these symptoms. The Chief of Vascular Surgery at Johns Hopkins Hospital, Dr. Melville William, I said I had 'tarsal tunnel syndrome', and that maybe you could help me."

"Yes, Jacob, I will try to help you. But you have a rare problem, and in truth, I have never operated on this problem before, so let me do a little reading* and research into Tarsal Tunnel Syndrome. Come back in a few weeks and we can make a plan together," I replied.

Jacob came back to see me. "Jacob," I said, "when a person has symptoms related to carpal tunnel syndrome, there is usually a place where the doctor can tap over the nerve, and if the nerve is compressed, the patient feels a tingling sensation go out into the fingers. This is called a 'positive Tinel sign, after a French doctor. It was also described by a German doctor, Doctor Hoffman. They both identified this sign working with injured soldiers from World War I, and described this sign in 1918. Let me see what happens when I tap on the tibial nerve in the tarsal tunnel region of your ankle."

"Doctor Dellon, when you tap there, I do get a sensation into the bottom of my foot and it goes out towards my toes," replied Jacob after I tapped on his ankle.

The Tarsal-Tunnel Syndrome

BY CAPTAIN CHARLES KECK, *Medical Corps, United States Army*

From the United States Army Hospital, Fort Hood, Texas

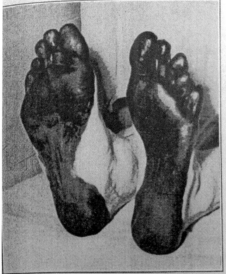

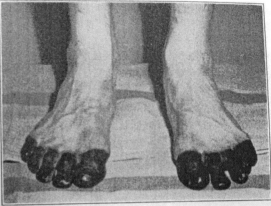

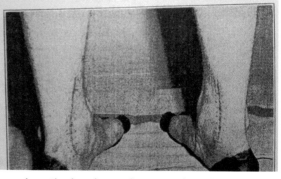

FIG. 1-B

FIG. 1-A

Figs. 1-A, 1-B, and 1-C: The distribution of complete anesthesia is indicated in black. Note in Fig. 1-C the extent of the operative incision for decompression of the posterior tibial nerve in the tarsal tunnel.

Figure 2-19. Photos of one of the first patients described with numbness and tingling in the darkly colored portions of the feet. This is one of the first papers to describe tarsal tunnel syndrome, which Doctor Keck, the author of the paper* described as being the carpal tunnel syndrome of the foot. The length of the incisions for the decompression surgery is seen in the lower right. Note they come quite high on the leg and not too far past the ankle. It was recommended that the foot be immobilized for 3 weeks to permit healing. The patient should not walk on the foot during that time, but use crutches. (With permission of the publisher.)

*Keck, C., Tarsal-Tunnel Syndrome, J. of Bone and Joint Surgery, 44A: 180-182, 1962.

"Jacob, this is very good news! I have been studying this problem. In the hand, there is just one tunnel that compresses the median nerve in the carpal tunnel. The location of the surgery described for tarsal tunnel surgery does not correspond with the location of the carpal tunnel in the hand. In fact, the tarsal location in the foot is actually the area of the wrist, the end of the forearm. I have identified the exact location for the compression of the nerves that go to the foot and toes and small muscles of the foot. There are actually four separate tunnels to release. I have designed an operation that combines two of these tunnels into one larger one, and I believe that this will relieve your foot symptoms from compression on the nerves."

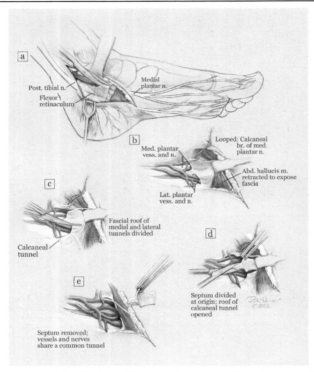

Figure 2-20. Dellon approach to the tarsal tunnel decompression. Four medial ankle tunnels are decompressed instead of just the one tarsal tunnel. In A) the white tissue is the covering of the tarsal tunnel. This is release to identify the important nerve patterns and the blood vessels within the tarsal tunnel itself, even though this large tunnel is usually NOT the site of pressure. In B), one of the foot muscles is retracted to show the roof of the tunnels with the most pressure upon the nerves, the medial and lateral plantar tunnels. In C and D) each of these tunnels is released, and in D) the tunnel to the nerve to the heel, the calcaneal nerve is also released. In E) the divider of the two tunnels is removed to create one large space for the nerves to travel in, completing the decompression. (With permission http://www.dellon.com)

My operation on Jacob for his tarsal tunnel syndrome began an enduring fascination with the nerve problems in the lower extremity. Today my approach to decompressing the four medial ankle tunnels is becoming the standard for treating this problem. As my new brochure, *Tarsal Tunnels Syndrome* (go to Dellon.com, and click on BROCHURES in the banner at the top of the page), makes clear even by its very name, it is critical to decompress each of these four tunnels to get relief of the foot and toe symptoms related to tibial nerve compression.

My approach to the other major nerve pathway in the leg, the peroneal nerve, has incorporated several important concepts. First, for the site of

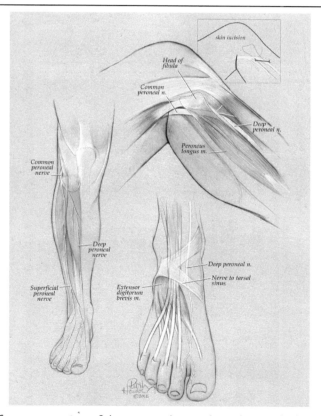

Figure 2-21. Sites for compression of the peroneal nerve branches in the knee, leg and foot. Incision to decompress the common peroneal nerve at the knee is shown in the upper right. The white covering of the muscles crossing this nerve cause compression of the nerve against the underlying the bone, the fibula. The deep peroneal nerve, in the lower right of this figure, is compressed against the underlying toe bones by an extra tendon. This tendon is removed. It is less common for the superficial peroneal nerve to become compressed on the outside of the leg, but this nerve, too, can be decompressed. (with permission http://www.Dellon.com)

compression at the knee, not only is the commonly opened connective tissue covering of the muscle that crosses the nerve released, but also, fibrous bands deep to that muscle, and fibrous bands deep to the nerve. This nerve at the knee is called the common peroneal nerve because it spits into one closer to the skin the lower part of the leg, the superficial peroneal nerve, and one beneath the muscles of the leg until it exits at the ankle, the deep peroneal nerve. In 1990, I described a site of compression for the deep peroneal nerve over the top of the foot.* This is a common site for nerve compression in patients with neuropathy, as is the site at the knee. Recently, the site of compression of the superficial peroneal nerve has been emphasized too. This less common site must be evaluated during the examination of the leg.

"Doctor Dellon, you helped my hands, can you help my feet?"

I used to say, "You had a nerve compression in your hands, but you have neuropathy in your feet, and a surgeon cannot operate on neuropathy." Now I say, "Let me examine your feet. If I find evidence of nerve entrapment at known sites of narrowing, then you also have nerve compressions here just as you did in your hands. When these nerve entrapments are in the legs, it gives you symptoms similar if not the same as neuropathy. If you have the most common three areas for nerve entrapments in your legs, at the outside of the knee, at the top of the foot, and on the inside of the ankle, then a Dellon Triple Nerve Decompression surgery has an excellent chance of helping your feet."

"Wonderful news Doctor Dellon. There is hope for me. But I am still a little confused. I am a diabetic. Will I still have neuropathy?"

---

*Dellon AL: Entrapment of the deep peroneal nerve on the dorsum of the foot. Foot and Ankle 11:73-80, 1990.

"Yes," I reply, "and that is a confusing problem. The metabolic problems created by diabetes do keep the nerve from working properly, but I have found that without the sites of anatomic narrowing compressing the nerves, that is, when surgery relieves the pressure on the nerves, even though the nerve still has the diabetic metabolic abnormalities within it, YOU will have your symptoms relieved. This is because for many people, the symptoms are due to compression of the nerves."

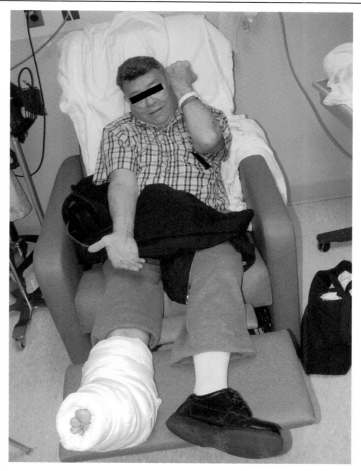

Figure 2-22. This man shows his wrist, forearm and elbow to demonstrate that he has already had relief of symptoms of nerve compressions in both of his arms. Some of the incisions have been outlined with a pen for visibility. He is diabetic with neuropathy. He is shown here with the bandage on his foot in the recovery room following a Dellon Triple Nerve Decompression to treat multiple nerve compressions in his right leg. The large dressing is placed to help him walk immediately after surgery using a walker. This allows the nerve to glide so they do not become entrapped again.

"Doctor Dellon, you helped my hands, and now you have also helped my feet. Thank you very much." People who have all 4 extremities decompressed for symptoms of nerve entrapments I like to call "QUADS."

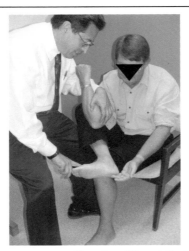

Figure 2-23. Doctor Dellon examines one of his first "Quads" who volunteers now to answer the Dellon Institutes "Diabetes Hotline" and its email "Pain Help Hotline" He is now eight years since his nerve decompressions in the year 1998.

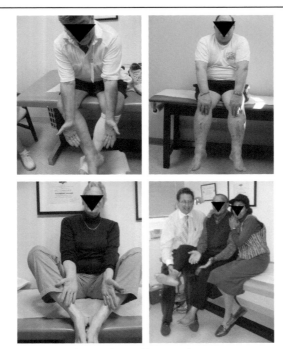

Figure 2-24. Four more patients who had a Dellon Triple Nerve Decompression in each of their four extremities, making them each a "Quad." The concepts that work for nerve compressions in the arm and hand work also in the leg and foot.

"How Long will it Take, and How Long will it Last?"

These are natural questions to ask:

"Doctor, Dellon, if I have the Triple Nerve Decompression surgery, how long will it take for me to know if the surgery really worked, and how will the results last?"

Usually when I am asked, "How long will it take?" I often reply, "Do you want me to rush?"

Usually when I am asked, "How long will it take to recover from surgery?" I often answer, "I rest about 10 or 15 minutes and then begin another operation."

Believe it or not, the patient usually laughs and relaxes a little bit.

The most common questions asked by patients with neuropathy are:

Q1) "Am I a good candidate for this surgery?" which I translate as asking "What are my chances for success?" and

Q2) "How long will it take for me to recover from my surgery?" which I translate as asking "When will my pain be gone and when will I get feeling back into my feet?" and

Q3) "How long will the results of the surgery last?" which I translate as asking "If I get good results, will my pain and numbness come back again?"

Let us give the answers by the numbers above:

ANSWER 1) CHANCE OF SUCCESS?

When I evaluate a patient with neuropathy, I am trying to decide if there is a place where a nerve is compressed. I tap along the nerve at the sites where compression can occur, demonstrated in Figure 9-25. When I tap on this site, if there is either pain or tingling going into the area of the symptoms, this is interpreted as being a "positive Tinel sign."

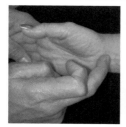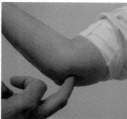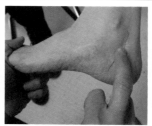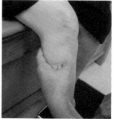

Figure 2-25. Examples of how I test for a local site of nerve compression in the patient with neuropathy. This is called the Tinel-Hoffman sign or simply, a positive Tinel sign.

If there is a positive Tinel sign, then your chance of having success with nerve decompression surgery, which is relief of symptoms, is at least 80%.*

ANSWER 2) HOW LONG TILL I KNOW IF THE SURGERY IS WORKING?

Each patient with neuropathy is tested with the Pressure-Specified Sensory Device™ (PSSD).

This measures sensibility in the skin and relates to your symptoms. Traditional, usually painful electrodiagnostic testing does not correlate well with symptoms. A brochure about "PSSD" testing is available on our website at DellonInstitutes.com. In 1989, I invented this computer-assisted neurosensory testing device with an aerospace engineer to help measure peripheral nerve function in the presence of neuropathy. The PSSD gives better information than those little nylon filaments, called Semmes-Weinstein monofilaments, and

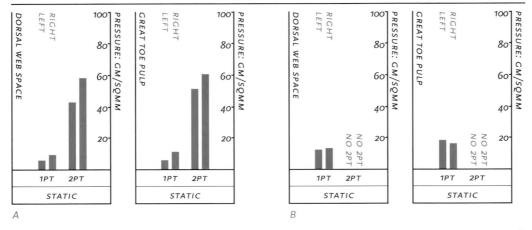

Figure 2-26. Neurosensory testing with the Pressure-Specified Sensory Device™ is demonstrated for a patient with neuropathy. The red color is the right and blue color is the left side of the body. The dorsal web is the top of the foot (peroneal nerve) and the great toe pulp is the big toe (tibial nerve). Higher numbers require more pressure and indicate a worse degree of nerve problems. When the red and blue bars are abnormal for both the peroneal (top of the foot) and the tibial nerve (the bottom of the foot), then the PSSD test results documents neuropathy as it does in both A and B. In A), the patient can still distinguish one from two static points, although not at normal levels of pressure and distance. With this degree of nerve damage, and the presence of a positive Tinel sign, the patient can expect to recover sensibility by 3 months after surgery. In B), with complete loss of two-point discrimination, more nerve fibers have died, and recovery from the Dellon Triple Nerve Decompression procedures may take up to one year to recover.

*Lee C, Dellon AL: Prognostic ability of Tinel sign in determining outcome for decompression surgery decompression surgery in diabetic and non-diabetic neuropathy, Annals of Plastic Surgery, 53:523-27, 2004

better information than measurements with vibration** in predicting who will develop an ulceration. These measurements, illustrated in Figure 2-26, document that neuropathy is present, and measure the degree of nerve damage present. If you have a moderately severe degree of nerve damage (Figure 2-26A) you should know that you are recovering from the Dellon Triple Nerve Decompression by 3 months after surgery. If the damage is more severe (Figure 2-26B) you have lost more nerve fibers: recovery can take up to one year.

ANSWER 3) HOW LONG WILL THE GOOD RESULTS FROM SURGERY LAST?

My first surgical procedures to restore sensation and relieve pain in diabetics with neuropathy and nerve compression began in 1982, and I have been able to keep in contact with some of my patients for a very long time. For example Figure 2-7 shows the foot of a patient that had the Dellon Triple Nerve Decompression 15 years earlier, with enough sensation preserved to prevent ulceration and amputation in the operated leg. Another long-term follow-up example is given in Figure 2-27.

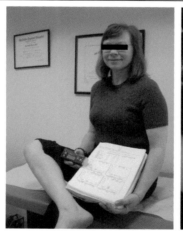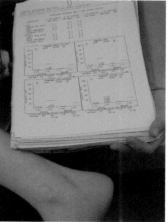

Figure 2-27. A Type I diabetic who had the Dellon Triple Nerve Decompression about 17 years ago. She holds her insulin pump in her right hand, and her most recent PSSD report in her left hand. The test demonstrates excellent sensibility in her feet. She has done a great job in maintaining her blood sugar level, and has not had any return of her neuropathy foot symptoms. She is a Registered Nurse and a Certified Diabetes Educator.

**Radoiu H, Rosson GD, Andonian G, Senatore J, Dellon AL: Comparison of measures of large-fiber nerve function in patients with chronic nerve compression and neuropathy, Journal of the American Podiatric Medical Association, 95: 438-445, 2005

"Doctor Dellon, is there somewhere I can look on the internet to learn the results of your surgery?" asked a thoughtful patient.

"Go to *NeuropathyRegistry.com*" I answered. A prospective, multi-center study group put this data on the internet as a public service of the

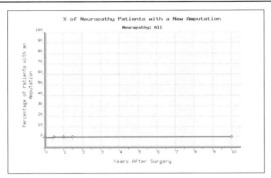

Figure 2-28. As of August 1, 2007, the limbs of 1494 patients have been operated on and there have been just 2 amputations instead of the predicted 38. 410 of these patients have had the Dellon Triple Nerve Decompression done in both legs. NeuropathyRegistry.com

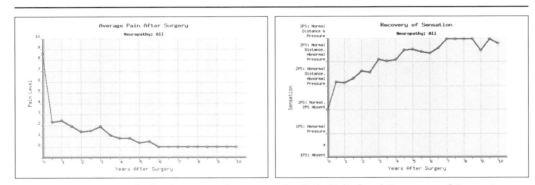

Figure 2-29. NeuropathyRegistry.com Outcomes for Pain Relief and Recovery of Sensation from August 1, 2007. Left: Most patients, before surgery, have a pain level of 8.5 out of 10.0 with ten being the worst pain ever experienced. By 6 months after a Dellon Triple Nerve Decompression, the average pain level is reduced to just 2 out or 10. This level of relief is maintained for many years. This graph contains 1172 patients. Right: Most patients, before surgery, have lost most ability to discriminate two points touching their big toe. Sensation recovers more slowly then relief of pain, but the graph demonstrates a steady recovery of sensation in these 1500 patients. Sensation remains improved for years.

Diabetic Neuropathy Foundation of the Southwest." Examples of Outcomes for Pain, Sensation, Ulcers and Amputations are given in Figures 2-28, 2-29, and 2-30.

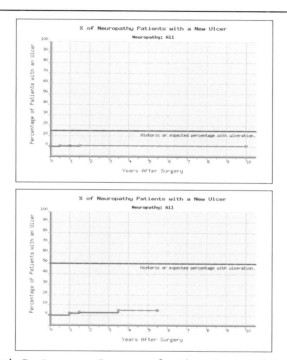

Figure 2-30. NeuropathyRegistry.com Outcomes for Ulceration as of August 1, 2007. Top: In diabetics with neuropathy, who have NOT had a previous ulceration, it is expected that one out of six (16%) will develop an ulceration of the foot or toe (red line). Among 1445 legs that had a Dellon Triple Nerve Decompression surgery, just 0.3% have had an ulceration. Bottom: In diabetics who have already had one ulceration that healed, it is expected that 50 to 60% will have that ulcer come back again or get a new ulceration (red line). Among 48 legs that had a history of a previous ulceration, and that then had a Dellon Triple Nerve Decompression, just 5.8% at 5.5 years developed a new ulceration, again demonstrating this surgery can change the history of diabetic neuropathy.

"Why Do Diabetics Get So Many Nerve Compressions" & "Why Does Your Surgery Work?"

As many times as I have answered these questions by patients and as many times as I have written about this subject, I still often feel as if the answer I going to give, again, now is just too simple to be believed. And yet this is the true answer:

When sugar, the molecule, glucose, goes into the nerve to give the nerve energy to create a nerve impulse and carry a message "upstream" to the brain or "downstream" to the fingers or toes, the glucose is changed into another sugar called sorbitol. You know that sugar dissolves easily into coffee and tea. The sorbitol inside the nerve pulls water into the nerve causing water to collect. This makes the nerve itself swell. The nerves in diabetics are swollen. When a nerve swells in a tight or narrow area, as it does when it passes across the elbow, or around the side of the knee, or into the wrist or the ankle, then the nerve comes under pressure. This pressure causes blood to flow more slowly in the nerve. This decreases the oxygen in the nerve. The response to decreased oxygen in the nerve is the numbness and tingling. With time, nerve fibers do not conduct their impulses as fast, and with further time, the nerve fibers actually die. The large nerve itself can become stuck to the sides of the tunnel.

There are other factors in diabetes that make the nerve susceptible to compression. One of these is that the sugar, the glucose, sticks to the connective tissues within the nerve, to make the nerve more stiff, so it does not glide as easily. This makes the nerve more likely to get in trouble if it is stretched. Also, this process narrows the tunnels through which the nerve travels.

Finally, we know that within the nerve fiber there is something similar to railroad tracks, called tubulin, along which the building blocks, the proteins for example, travel from the cell body near the spinal cord, to the fingers and toes. In diabetes, the speed at which this transport system works is slowed down. When the building blocks, the proteins, cannot be delivered to the compressed sites along the nerve in the tight tunnels, then the nerve cannot repair itself properly.

This combination of metabolic processes is the underlying cause for the nerves in the diabetic to be susceptible to compression.

In my approach, these metabolic processes are NOT changed. Rather the tight regions of nerve compression are opened. All patients with diabetic neuropathy are NOT operated on. Patients with nerve compression at known sites of compression will be a candidate for the Dellon Triple Nerve Decompression. It is that simple.

Idiopathic Neuropathy

"Doctor Dellon," said Jerry, "No one knows why I have neuropathy. My feet burn, sometimes like they are on fire, and sometimes they just feel heavy and dead. I do not have diabetes, will your surgery work for me?"

"Jerry, you are in great shape, and do not have diabetes, and probably will not get diabetes either. The American Neuropathy Associates estimates that there are as many people in America with neuropathy of unknown cause, or idiopathic neuropathy, as there are diabetics with neuropathy. The good news, Jerry, is that 'Yes!,'" my approach to neuropathy also works very well for people exactly like you."

"Jerry," I continued, "many types of neuropathy create a condition where the nerve becomes very likely to become compressed. In diabetes, the sugar pulls water into the nerve, making it swell. As the nerve in the diabetic increases in size, it gets compressed in areas that are normally tight in the arms and legs. This susceptibility to compression can happen to you too, even though we may not understand what the exact mechanism is. You have had a skin biopsy that shows your small nerve fibers, related to pain and temperature perception, are dying, but your neurosensory testing you had with the Pressure-Specified Sensory Device™ demonstrated that your large fiber nerves, the ones related to touch and pressure sensations, are also dying. You do not have a small fiber neuropathy, but a mixed fiber neuropathy, which is quite common. So I am going to examine your legs and feet to see if we can find any sites of compression of your nerves.

Not all patients make as great a recovery as Jerry did. (See Figure 2-31.) Some patients have either continued pain, or, in some unusual cases more pain as the nerves regenerate. Nerves regenerate at one inch per month. During this painful period, some patients believe they are either not getting better or perhaps their nerve has been injured. It is therefore usual to repeat the PSSD test to document that nerve regeneration is

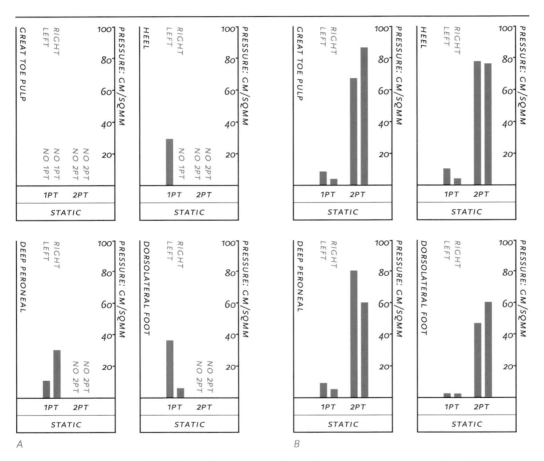

A   B

Figure 2-31. A: This man has idiopathic neuropathy with nerve compression in both legs. Note the absent blue (left leg) and red (right leg) bars related to 1PT and 2PT, demonstrating a severe degree of neuropathy with nerve fiber death. B: This test is repeated two years after the second leg had its Dellon Triple Nerve Decompression surgery. His pain is greatly relieved and he has recovered sensation as shown in the PSSD print outs, demonstrating recovery to almost normal levels of the bars for both feet for each nerve decompressed.

occurring. Another example of neuropathy improvement is documented by the PSSD test is in Figure 9-32.

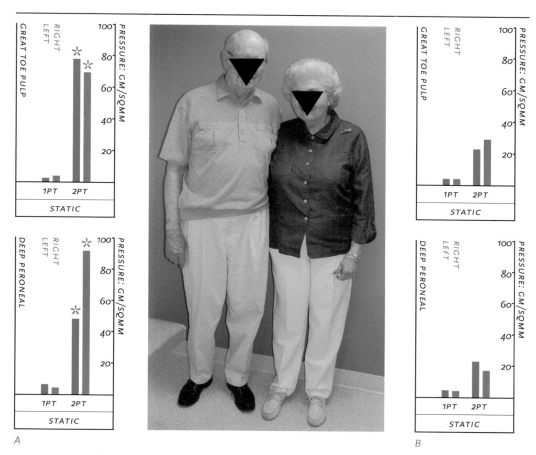

Figure 2-32. A: The woman is one year after having a Dellon Triple Nerve Decompression for idiopathic neuropathy on both legs. Her neuropathy was not as advanced as that demonstrated by the PSSD test in Figure 2-31. A: Prior to surgery, note that the bars for the left leg (blue) and for the right leg (red) are still present, but have an asterisk (*) on top of them indicating that the nerve fibers are dying. B: At one year after surgery, note that the height of the bars has diminished to almost normal levels and there is no longer an * present, demonstrating that the nerves have regenerated. This patient has improved faster than the one in Figure 2-31 because the degree of nerve compression was not as advanced. NERVE RECOVERY IS FASTER IN SOMEONE WHOSE NERVES ARE AT AN EARLIER STAGE OF COMPRESSION. THE PSSD TEST CAN IDENTIY THE NERVE COMPRESSION AND NEUROPATHY AT THE EARLIEST STAGE.*

*Radoiu H, Rosson GD, Andonian G, Senatore J, Dellon AL: Comparison of measures of large-fiber nerve function in patients with chronic nerve compression and neuropathy, Journal of American Podiatric Medical Association, 95: 438-445, 2005.

Chemotherapy Neuropathy

"Doctor Dellon I survived ovarian cancer only to become a painful prisoner to my feet. They hurt so much I cannot get around much," Nancy said describing her current situation. She went on, "Doctor Dellon, the Cisplatin drug they gave me was a miracle. My cancer has been gone now for 4 years. I am a cancer survivor…but a neuropathy cripple! I love to ski and am a Ski Patrol member, but I have no balance and cannot ski anymore. I work inspecting ski lifts, but I have been disabled now for four years due to my neuropathy. Can your work with diabetic neuropathy patients be used to help me?"

"Yes, Nancy, there is hope for you," I told her.*

My research into chemotherapy neuropathy was begun after my work with diabetes. In the diabetes research I learned that there were problems in diabetes that made the nerve more likely to become compressed. This is also true for some chemotherapy drugs (see Table 9-1).

Table 2-1.

Vincristine	Taxol	Cisplatin	Thalidimide

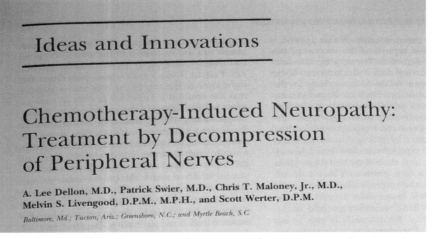

Figure 2-33. Title page of the first report of treatment of nerve compression in patients with chemotherapy-induced neuropathy, reported in 2004.

*Dellon AL, Swier P, Levingood M, Maloney CT: Cisplatin/Taxol neuropathy: Treatment by decompression of peripheral nerve. Plast Reconstr Surg, 114:478-483, 2004.

"Nancy," I continued to explain, "in the hands and feet, the tight tunnels the nerves pass through at the elbow and knee, and at the wrist and ankle can create sites of compression even in a normal nerve. In the patient who has chemotherapy, some forms of the drugs attach inside the nerve and make the nerves more likely to get compressed. Surgery can release these nerves, relieve your pain and restore your sensation. Your balance may return as well."

"Doctor Dellon, doctors helped me beat my cancer, and I want you to help me beat my neuropathy. Schedule the surgery for my first leg."

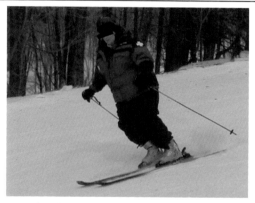

Figure 2-34. Nancy, one year after having the Dellon Triple Nerve Decompression on her second leg. Her balance restored, her pain relieved, she is back skiing again. She says, "I AM A CANCER SURVIVOR AND I HAVE BEATEN NEUROPATHY TOO."

"Doctor Dellon, what did my nerve look," asked Stanley, a man who had not felt his foot for two years.

"Stanley," I answered him, "you are the first person with chemotherapy-induced neuropathy from Thalidomide. The drug has helped your multiple myeloma cancer to stop growing, but it also has given you a painful neuropathy leaving your with numbness too. Stanley, I took a photograph of the nerve on the outside of your knee, the common peroneal nerve. The nerve had a straight line across it at the site of compression by fibrous bands. You were born with the bands. The chemotherapy made the nerve sensitive to pressure, giving you your symptoms." See Figure 2-35.

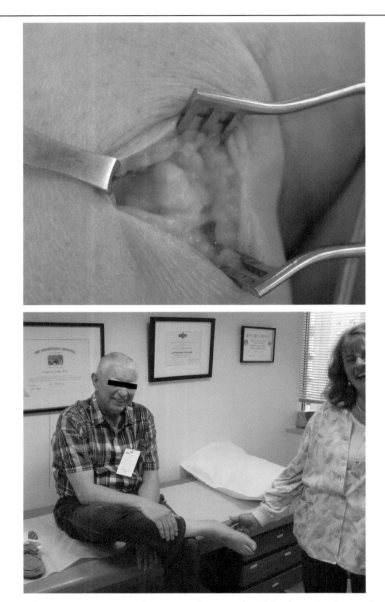

Figure 2-35. Top: The common peroneal nerve at the outside of the knee is shown during surgery. The flattened part of the nerve is noted. The normally white nerve is now slightly yellow due to the chemotherapy, and swollen where it entered the tight area. This nerve goes to the top of the foot (compare to other views of common peroneal nerve, Fig 1-12). Bottom: 2 weeks after a Dellon Triple Nerve Decompression, the bottom of the foot is tickled by Rita Moore in Doctor Dellon's office. Note the patient laughing as he can now feel his foot. The tibial nerve and its branches in the inside of the ankle were released too, restoring sensation to the bottom of the foot.

Heavy Metal Poisoning

Eat too much tuna fish? You could have mercury poisoning. Are you a plumber, a welder, a sand blaster? You could have lead poisoning. Arsenic poisoning may give you neuropathy before it kills you!

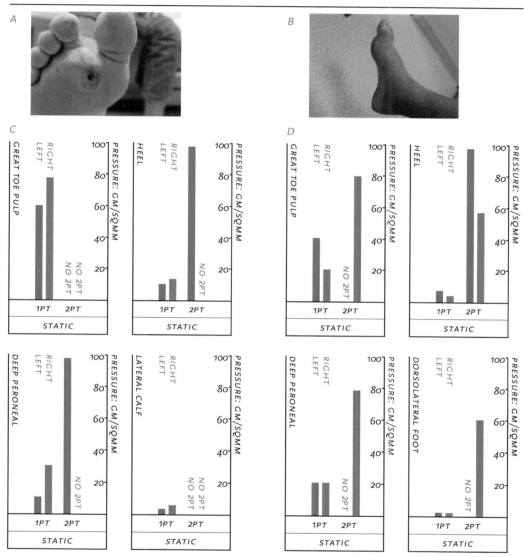

Figure 2-36. Example of Arsenic Poisoning. The severe sensory loss has resulted in an ulceration (A) and skin dryness and cracking (B), similar to that seen in a diabetic. The first neurosensory testing with the PSSD demonstrated severe neuropathy in both the right (red bars) and the left (blue bars) (C). In D) 3 months after a Dellon Triple Nerve Decompression on the right leg, note the PSSD demonstrates a nerve regeneration pattern on the right side, with increased numbers of red bars in the regeneration pattern for each nerve decompressed (peroneal and tibial), while the left (blue bars), non-operated side, remains without improvement.

Lead poisoning was the first neuropathy to be studied experimentally. It is known that the lead causes the attachments of the cells that line the blood vessels to separate, and fluid from the blood vessels leaks out through the walls of the blood vessels. When this happens to the blood vessels in the nerves, fluid enters the nerve causing the nerve to swell. Therefore, just like in the diabetic, the nerve in the patient with heavy metal poisoning is swollen. This makes the nerve more likely to be come compressed in the tight tunnels. The Dellon Triple Nerve Decompression therefore can be effective in patients with heavy metal poisoning who also have nerve compressions.

The "heavy metals" are electronically like calcium, and have a positive charge. They are therefore absorbed and stored in the bone, and can remain there, slowly coming out over time to keep the levels in the blood high, and continuing to give you symptoms.

A laboratory test, called a heavy metal toxicity screening test, can identify if these metals are present in the blood. There are treatments that can remove these heavy metals from your body, and certainly this treatment, called "chelation therapy" should be tried first.

Leprosy

"Doctor Dellon, I have read of your work with patients who have diabetes and neuropathy. I am in charge of the Father Damien House in Guyaquil, Ecuador. We take care of people with Leprosy, which, as you know, is also called Hansen's Disease. Doctor Dellon, even when my patients have been treated by antibiotics, and the bacteria that caused their leprosy is killed, my patients continue with numbness in the hands and feet, weakness in their hands and legs, and many also have pain. Doctor Dellon," said Sister Annie, "can your approach to nerves help my patients? Can your approach lessen or prevent their disabilities?"

"Yes Sister Annie," I answered her, "There is real hope for them."

"Sister Annie," I continued. "This is a historic day. We are here because one of my students, Dr. James Wilton, from New Hampshire, has organized this medical mission. He is a Podiatric foot and ankle surgeon. He knows well my work with restoring sensation and preventing deformity in diabetics. I told Dr. Wilton about Dr. Paul Brand's pioneering work in Leprosy in India in the 1940's and 1950's, in which he demonstrated that the loss of tissue in leprosy was due to loss of sensitivity. He demonstrated that the nerves become involved close to joints. I suggested to Dr. Wilton that my work with diabetics could be transferred to leprosy patients. Just as you have said, the bacteria that cause leprosy are treated well now with antibiotics. But the bacteria attach to nerves in regions of the nerves close to the skin, and the body's reaction to the bacteria cause the nerve to swell. I believe that the progressive deformity in leprosy is due to chronic nerve compression, and that the operative approach I have developed for diabetic nerve entrapments will work in leprosy."

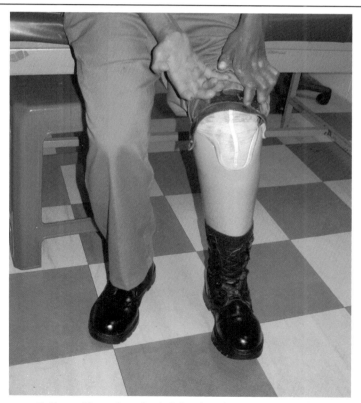

Figure 2-37. Leprosy Patient. Note that the left leg has been amputated due to ulceration resulting from loss of sensation, similar to what occurs in the diabetic with neuropathy. Note the hand deformities due to bilateral median and ulnar nerve compressions, not Leprosy.

In July of 2004, Dr Wilton, and David Seiler, who is the Director of Neurosensory Training for the Dellon Institutes for Peripheral Nerve Surgery®, made a survey trip to the Father Damien Foundation in Guyaquil, Ecuador to do neurosensory testing and physical examinations on patients who had been treated with antibiotics for leprosy but who still had symptoms in the hands and feet, and had progressive disability. David Seiler and I have worked together in research since 1982.

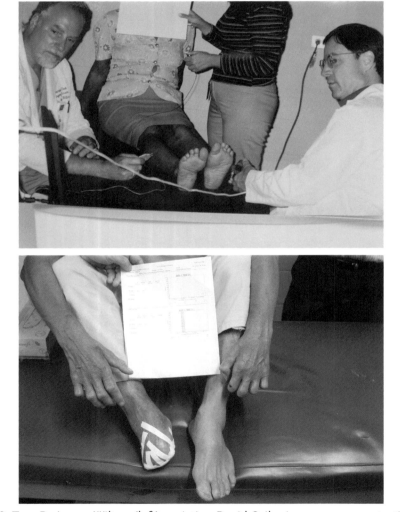

Figure 2-38. Top: Dr James Wilton (left) assisting David Seiler in neurosensory testing with the Pressure-Specified Sensory Device™ in Guyaquil, Ecuador, July 2004. Bottom: A patient with his PSSD test result. Note the amputated right toes and left fingers due to loss of sensation. Would appropriate nerve decompression earlier have prevented this?

My approach to nerve problems in leprosy followed from my approach to nerve problems in the diabetic.

The double crush concept implies that one site of compression predisposes a nerve to a second site of compression. A metabolic problem like diabetes could be the first "crush." In leprosy, the attachment of the bacteria could be the first "crush." Then each other site along the nerve needed to be decompressed. So for the median nerve in the upper extremity, decompression needed to be done at the wrist and the forearm, for the ulnar nerve at the wrist and the forearm. While historically, surgeons had tried to decompress the ulnar nerve at the elbow, my approach included the submuscular transposition, described in Chapter 1, plus an internal neurolysis of the ulnar nerve at the elbow, and the neurolysis of the ulnar nerve at the wrist at the same time. Furthermore, at the wrist, the motor branch of the ulnar nerve was separately released. A similar approach was taken in the lower extremity.

In order to minimize the number of operations per patient, and to minimize their time under anesthesia, the plan was for Dr. Wilton to operate on a leg while I operated on an arm at the same time.

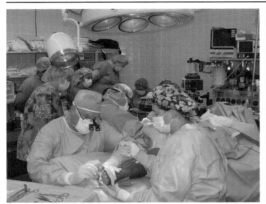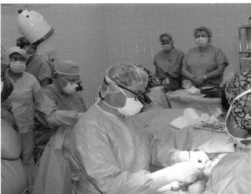

Figure 2-39. Left: The team operating in Ecuador for the first time. Note Dr. Wilton, green hat, operating on the foot in the lower left, with Dr. Dellon directly behind him operating on the right arm. Dellon Triple Nerve Decompressions were done in the arm and in the leg. Right: Another patient, with Dr. Dellon in foreground operating on the left elbow, and Dr. Wilton behind Doctor Dellon, doing a Dellon Triple Nerve Decompression.

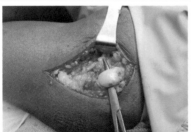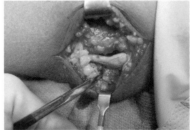

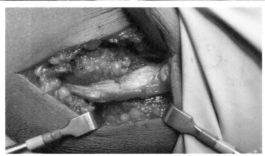

Figure 2-40. Ulnar nerve decompression in a patient with leprosy. Top left: Note the huge size of the ulnar nerve above the elbow. Top right: After release of the cubital tunnel, in which the ulnar nerve is compressed behind the elbow, note the narrow area of nerve compression. Bottom: After mircrosurgical neurolysis of the ulnar nerve. The nerve was then transposed into a submuscular position using Dellon musculofascial lengthening technique.

The first surgical expedition to apply this approach to leprosy was in November 2004.

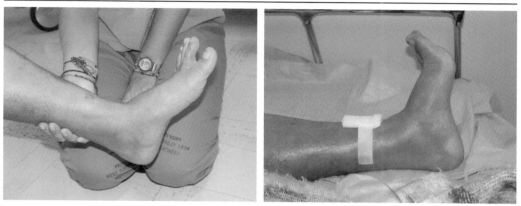

Figure 2-41. Leprosy patient with a peroneal nerve palsy. Left: Prior to surgery, the patient could not lift up his foot or his big toe. Right: In the recovery room, right after decompression of the common peroneal nerve at the knee, the patient can now lift up his foot and extend his big toe. This is a reversal of a paralyzed leg in this leprosy patient.

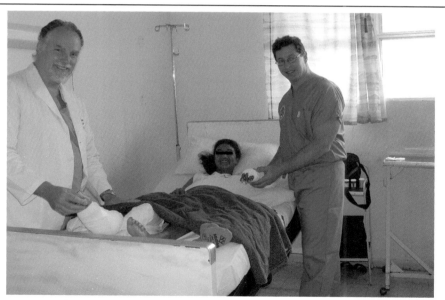

Figure 2-42. Dr Wilton, left, and Dr. Dellon, right, tickling the toes and the fingertips of this young woman with leprosy. She had a Dellon Triple Nerve Decompression on left hand and right leg. The day after surgery, she smiles as she can feel again.

The Dellon Institutes for Peripheral Nerve Surgery® has sent continued this work which has been sponsored by the Perfect World Foundation. In a subsequent trip, Dr. Scott Nickerson, an Orthopedic Surgeon (Figure 2-3), joined the trip with his wife to carry out an independent analysis of the surgical results. And Dr Christopher T. Maloney Jr, MD, a Plastic Surgeon, from Tucson, joined the mission with his father, Christopher T. Maloney Sr., MD, a retired Cardiac Surgeon. The most recent mission was in November 2006. The work is successful and continues.

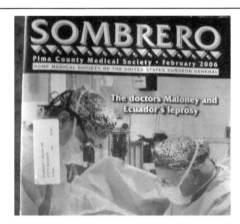

Figure 2-43. Dr. Christopher T. Maloney Jr., MD, a Plastic Surgeon from Tucson, and his father, a retired Cardiac Surgeon, operated together on the leprosy patients. They are shown here on the cover of the local medical society news.

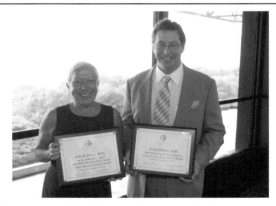

Figure 2-44. Dr. Julia Terzis, MD, PhD, left, and Dr. A. Lee Dellon, MD, right, with their awards from the Plastic Surgery Educational Foundation in 2005. Dr. Terzis received her award for work with obstetrical palsy, and Dr. Dellon for his work with leprosy. Both Dr. Terzis and Dr. Dellon have been President of the American Society for Peripheral Nerve, and of the American Society for Reconstructive Microsurgery

Communicating Success To Different Communities

In the most professional manner, it is critical to educate physicians and the public alike about out success relieving pain, restoring sensation, and preventing ulcers, infections, and amputations in those patients with neuropathy.

I have been trying to do this for more than 20 years.

May I tell you about the most important experimental work, which was published in the early 1990's? After making the observations that I could help my neuropathy patients if they had a nerve compression present, I studied this problem for 6 years in diabetic rats. What if there were a group of rats that did not have a site of compression, would they develop neuropathy as the diabetic rat usually did? Neuropathy in the rat is identified by measuring the rat's footprints after their feet have been put in water-based paint.

Figure 2-45. Dellon Institutes for Peripheral Nerve Surgery® logo includes the rat footprint, used to measure neuropathy experimentally, as a symbol of our continuing research and a reflection of our motto: "Being Academic in Private Practice™." There are three other icons in the logo. The PSSD is at the top, the book stands for scientific publications, and the loupes represent microsurgery.

Results of this study* can be seen in Figure 2-46.

Doing the same operation in rats that I did in my patients changed the natural history of diabetic neuropathy in this species of rat!

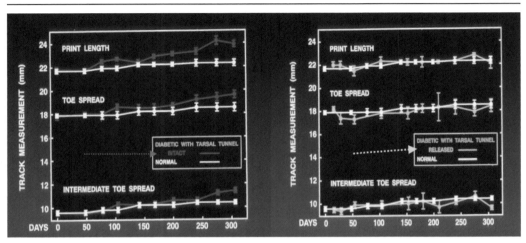

Figure 2-46. DIABETIC RATS WITHOUT A TARSAL TUNNEL DO NOT DEVELOP NEUROPATHY. Results of an experimental study in diabetic rats. Each rat has a blood sugar of 400. The study lasted for one year. The white lines are the measurements of the characteristics of the foot of a normal, non-diabetic rat. Left: The red lines are those same measurements in the diabetic rat with a tarsal tunnel. As the red lines separate from the white lines, it demonstrates that diabetic rats, with their normal tarsal tunnels, have a progressive, neuropathy and have trouble walking normally. Right: The yellow lines are those same measurements in diabetic rats who have no tarsal tunnel (they were released at the beginning of the study), and these diabetic rats have footprints that look just like the non-diabetic, normal (white line) rats. The diabetic rats without a tarsal tunnel, without a site of compression, did not develop neuropathy.

*Dellon ES, Dellon AL: Functional assessment of neurologic impairment: Track analysis in diabetic and compression neuropathies. Plastic Reconstrive Surgery 88:686-694, 1991
*Dellon ES, Dellon AL, Seiler WA IV: Effect of tarsal tunnel decompression in streptozotocin-induced diabetic rats. Microsurgery 15:265-268, 1994.

This is the story we must bring to people everywhere: THERE IS HOPE AND OPTIMISM FOR THE DIABETIC WITH SYMPTOMS OF NEUROPATHY IF THERE ARE COMPRESSED NERVES THAT CAN BE DECOMPRESSED WITH SURGERY.

To get the word out to the community, each patient who has been improved will speak to their doctors and friends to let them know there is now hope for them. I try to speak to groups in the community. Figure 2-48 is an example of this. I spoke for a retirement community to give them hope.

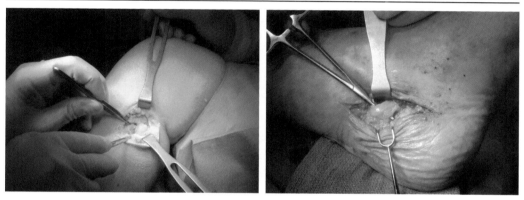

Figure 2-47: Diabetic with neuropathy Left: Note swollen yellow common peroneal nerve at knee entrapment site. Right: Note swollen yellow tibial nerve in the tarsal tunnel at entrapment site, crossing over the clamp. It is this swelling in the nerve that makes it so susceptible to nerve compression at these sites of anatomic narrowing. The areas of tightness can be opened in surgery, as shown above.

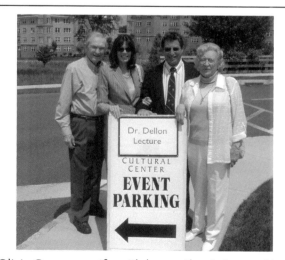

Figure 2-48. Luiann Olivia Greer, my wife, with her mother JoAnn and her father Jack Greer and myself at Willow Valley Retirement Community at the time of my lecture. More than 10% of people over the age of 65 will have neuropathy from one cause or another.

The goal of the United States of America for the year 2000 was to reduce the amputation rate by 40%. That goal was not met. Now it is the goal of Healthy Choice USA for 2010. (see amputation rates in Table 2-2).

We need to get the message out that if you have a Dellon Triple Decompression surgery, your rate of amputation will approach 0%.

Table 2-2.

AMPUTATION RATES 1994 (*per 1000 of population*)

African Americans	9.3
Caucasians	5.7
Male	10.9
Female	6.2
Under 64 years old	6.5
Between 65-74 years old	10.2
Over 74 years old	11.9
Hispanics	unkown
Native Americans	unknown

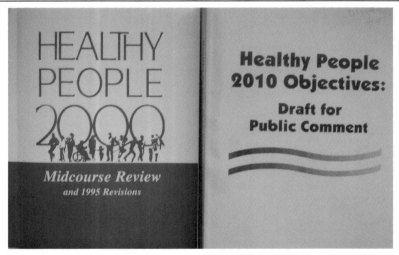

Figure 2-49. It is the stated goal for the United States of America to reduce the amputation rate by 40%. But there is no approach that has been successful so far except the approach that I have described here.

Public Service at Community Diabetic Expos

The Dellon Institute for Peripheral Nerve Surgery in Boston participated in 2005 in the Diabetes Expo sponsored by the American Diabetes Association. Free neurosensory testing of the feet of diabetics was done. (see Figure 2-50). In June of 2006, Doctor Dellon was invited to participate in the program of the American Diabetes Association annual meeting, in Washington, DC. A report is available on Dellon.com.

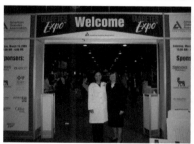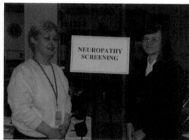

Figure 2-50. The Boston Dellon Institute is directed by Dr Virgina Hung, (left) with Vicki Muse, RN, CDE. Vicki and Gina Andonian, (right) came from the Dellon Institute in Baltiomore to do the neurosensory testing testing for Dr Hung in Boston.

The Native American Community

The amputation rate of the Native American community is probably the highest rate in the United States. It is somehow conveniently "unknown." In 1997, I went to the T'ohono Odham nation outside Tucson, Arizona at the request of the Podiatrist of the Indian Health Service in order to help them with this problem. Bringing help to people can be a challenging problem.

The biggest success has come with the Gila Reservation, between Tucson and Phoenix, where a group of very proactive Podiatrists, under the leadership of Wes Yamada, DPM have introduced neurosensory testing with the PSSD and have taken my Advanced Lower Extremity Peripheral Nerve Workshop, learning the technical skills necessary to do the Dellon Triple Decompression to their population of diabetics. It is the Gila reservation where the original distinction of Type I and Type II diabetics occurred.

In August of 2005, I spoke before the Association of American Indian Physicians in Washington, DC, and in July of 2006 at the Headquarters of the Indian Health Service in Rockville, Maryland. I am hopeful that soon the success of my work in other populations of diabetics can be duplicated on for the Native Americans.

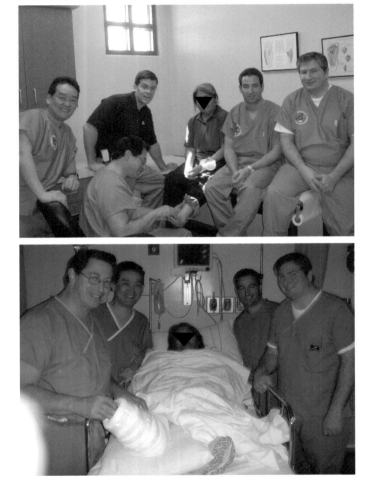

Figure 2-51. The first Native American diabetic patient from the Gila Reservation in Arizona at the University Medical Center of the University of Arizona. Top: She is being examined by me prior to surgery. In the black shirt, is Dr. Christopher T. Maloney, Jr, MD. Surrounding us are the Podiatric foot and ankle surgeons from the Gila Reservation from Sacaton, Arizona. Clockwise from the left: Wes Yamada, Wes Taxier, and Paul Keller. Bottom: In the recovery room immediately after the Dellon Triple Nerve Decompression on her right leg, the patient smiles as she can feel her foot again. Her group of Podiatrists from the Gila Reservation surround her.

The International Community

DOCTOR DELLON TRAINED SURGEONS WHO ARE PROVIDING PATIENTS WITH THIS SURGERY IN 18 COUNTRIES. SOME OF THESE DOCTORS ARE SHOWN HERE.

AUSTRIA

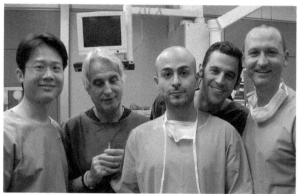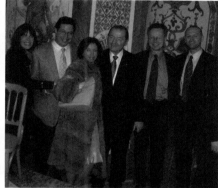

Figure 2-52. Left: Oskar Aszmann, MD, Associate Professor of Plastic Surgery at the University of Vienna (surgeon on the right end) is shown with his laboratory staff in 2006, and (right) with Doctor Hanno Millesi and his wife Dagmar, also a Plastic Surgeon, at Dr. Millesi's 2006 Symposium on Peripheral Nerve Surgery, at which Dr. Dellon (left with wife, Luiann) presented world results of the Dellon Triple Nerve decompression surgery. Dr. Aszmann is the pioneer to introduce this work into Austria. They are shown at a Mozart concert in the historic hall in which Mozart's music was originally played.

BRAZIL

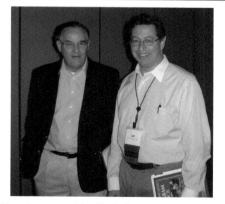

Figure 2-53. Marcus Castro Ferreira, MD, Chief of Plastic Surgery in Sao Paolo, Brazil, with Doctor Dellon at a meeting in 2005. Doctor Ferreira is his their country's pioneer in introducing the Dellon Triple Nerve Decompression surgery and neurosensory testing into his country.

ENGLAND

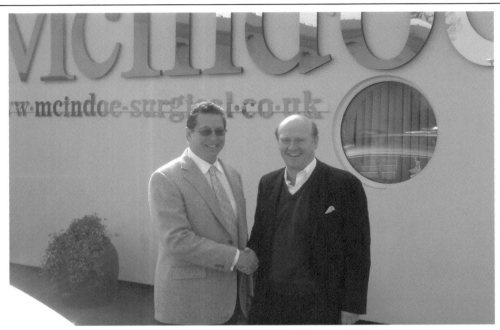

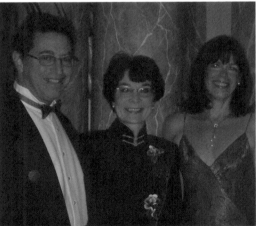

Figure 2-54. Top: Doctor Nicholas Parkhouse, the Plastic Surgeon in charge of the McIndoe Plastic Surgery Clinic in East Grinstead, United Kingdom, is the Director of the Dellon Institute for Peripheral Nerve Surgery in England. He is shown above with Dr. Dellon. Bottom: Doctor Sally Stevens is shown between Doctor Dellon and his wife Luiann in London, where she did her research on the evolution of the knee joint. They are at the Guild Hall honoring the Chinese New Year in January of 2006.

CHINA

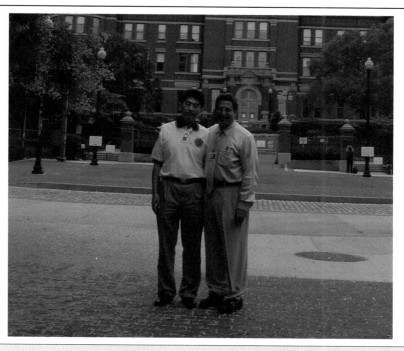

Figure 2-55. In 2005, Doctor Yong Yao, a neurosurgeon on the faculty of Peking Union Medical College in Beijing, came to the Baltimore to study with Doctor Dellon. Doctor Yong Yao is pictured standing with Doctor Dellon in front of the Johns Hopkins Hospital in Baltimore, where Doctor Dellon is a Professor of Plastic Surgery and Neurosurgery. Doctor Yong Yao began to do the Dellon Triple Nerve Decompression in China in the Department of Neurosurgery of Professor Wang. Their first publication of Dr. Yong Yao's results is shown above from the Nervous System and Mental Health Journal. In January of 2007, Dr. Yong Yao presented the results of his first 100 Dellon Triple Procedures at the American Society for Reconstructive Surgery meeting. Doctor Yong Yao is the Director of the Dellon Institute for Peripheral Nerve Surgery in China.

DUBAI

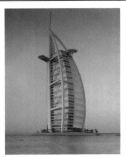
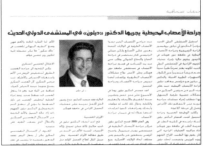
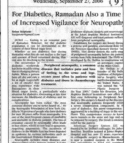
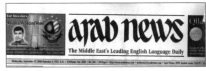

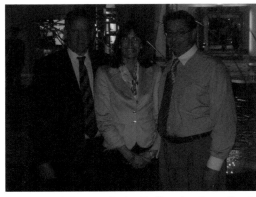
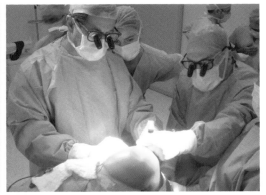

Figure 2-56. In 2006, the Dellon Institute for Peripheral Nerve Surgery opened in Dubai, United Arab Emirates. Articles appeared in the Dubai press. Lower left: Gordon Pincock, CEO of the Sulaiman Al-Habib Medical Group, Dubai, UAE, is shown with Doctor Dellon and his wife, Luiann. Lower right: Doctor John Bouillon, on the right, an Orthopedic surgeon who trained at Johns Hopkins with Doctor Dellon, is shown operating with Doctor Dellon at the International Modern Hospital in Duabi. Dr. Bouillon is the Director of the Dellon Institute in Dubai, where the Dellon Triple Nerve Decompression will be able to help the large Emirate population of diabetics. Under direction also of Dr. Bouillon and the Habib Medical Group, this surgery will be done at the American Surgical Center, the first outpatient surgical center in the region. The Dellon approach to peripheral nerve problems will soon be available in Abu Dhabi.

ITALY

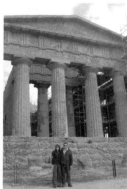
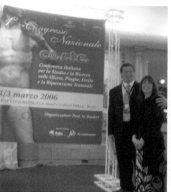
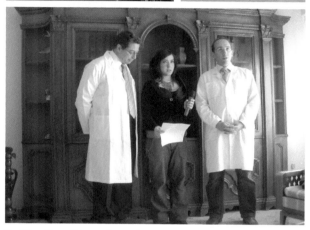

Figure 2-57. Top Left: The first Wound Healing meeting in Rome, directed by Dr. Professor Nicolò Scuderi, Chief of Plastic Surgery, University of Rome School of Medicine. Dr Dellon spoke on the Triple Nerve Decompression surgery preventing ulceration and amputation. Luiann is with him, March 1, 2006. Top right: Agrigento, Sicily, where Luiann and Lee identify with the reconstruction of the ancient ruins, just as his surgery can restore lost sensibility to the foot. Bottom: Doctor Fabio Quatra, a Plastic Surgeon who trained with Doctor Dellon, is interviewed for TV as he introduces the Dellon Institute for Peripheral Nerve Surgery to his city, Palermo, Sicily, where he will be its Director. Dr Fabio Quatra combined with Dr Dellon to write a chapter on "Decompression of Peripheral Nerves in Patients with Diabetic Neuropathy" for the first on-line electronic book on Plastic Surgery, edited by Fabio Santanelli and Nicolo Scuderi, "Chirurgia Plastica Ricostruttiva Ed Esthetica" from the University of Rome "La Spienza", published in Italian in June of 2007.

INDIA

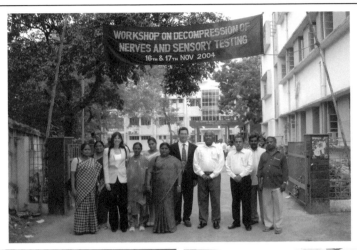

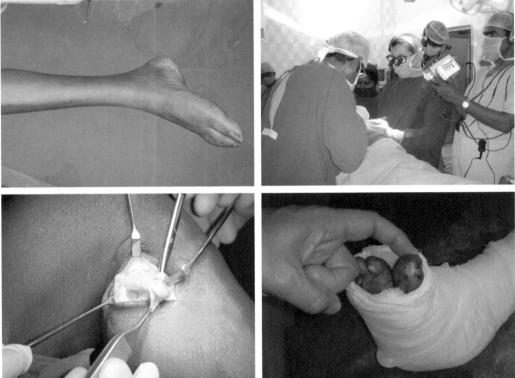

Figure 2-58. Top: Doctor Dellon teaching and operating in Chenai (Madras), India in 2004 at the invitation of Doctor G. Balakrishnan, Chief of Plastic Surgery at the Stanley Government Hospital (center next to Doctor Dellon). Center left: The paralyzed foot of a patient with leprosy. Center right: Doctors Dellon and Balakrishnan operating on this patient. Bottom left: The thickened and scarred peroneal nerve at the knee is decompressed. Bottom right: The next day, the patient can begin to lift up his big toe, as the paralysis reverses after the surgery.

INDIA

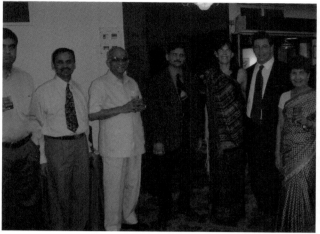
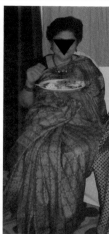
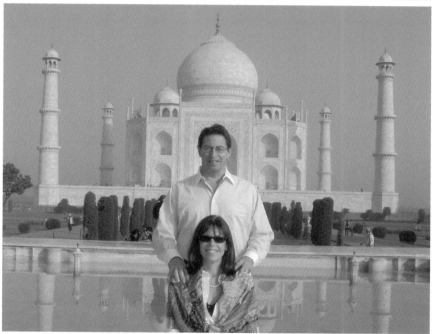

Figure 2- 59. Top left: In Mumbai (Bombay), India, at the invitation of Doctor Suresh Tambwekr, Chief of Plastic Surgery at Bombay Foundation Hospital, Doctor Dellon did his Triple Nerve Decompression surgery on a diabetic. Dr. Tambwekr (center in white) has been the leader to introduce this surgery into India, and has published one paper on his results. Top right: This woman came to the United States for Dr. Dellon to operate on both arms and both legs to treat her diabetic neuropathy related to nerve compression. She is at a reception honoring Dr. Dellon in Mumbai. Bottom: After Doctor Dellon spoke for the Indian Association of Plastic Surgery about his neuropathy work, in 2004, he and his wife, Luiann, visited the Taj Mahal in Agra, India. Across from the entrance to the Taj Mahal is a leporsarium.

TURKEY

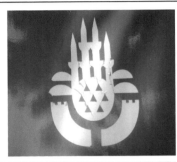

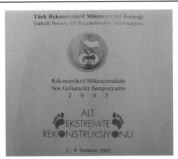

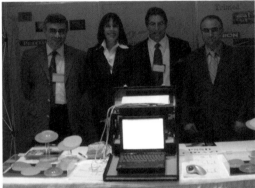

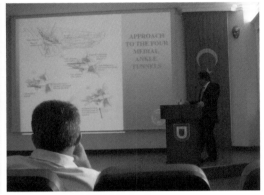

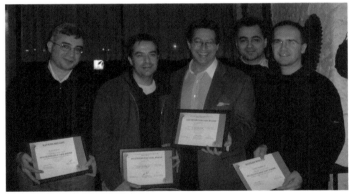

Figure 2-60. Dr Dellon spoke at the Turkish Society for Plastic and Reconstructive Micro-surgery, invited by Fuat Yuksel, MD, a Plastic Surgeon from Istanbul (city symbol, upper left). Upper right: Program cover for the meeting. Dr Yuksel, through his own research, confirmed Dr. Dellon's basic science and clinical research with the Triple Nerve Decompression for Diabetic Neuropathy. He is at left with the Dellons, as the Neurosensory testing device is displayed (center left) at the meeting and below, on the left, with Plastic Surgeons, Ferit Demirkan, Dr. Dellon, Yavuz Demir, and Alper Sari. Center right: Dr. Dellon giving his lecture at the meeting.

Pain Solutions Summary

Traditional medial teaching is that neuropathy is "progressive and irreversible," which means that if you have neuropathy you are not likely to get better. This is especially true for neuropathy in diabetics.

The NEWS is that through years of my research, which has now been confirmed by many other doctors throughout the world, we know that *in many patients with neuropathy the symptoms are due mostly to compression of nerves in the arms and legs, hands and feet.* The best news is that nerve compression sites can be decompressed surgically to remove the pressure on the nerves that are causing the symptoms.

IF YOU HAVE A NERVE COMPRESSION ASSOCIATED WITH YOUR NEUROPATHY, THEN YOU SHOULD HAVE AN 80% CHANCE TO RELIEVE PAIN AND RECOVER SENSATION BY NERVE DECOMPRESSION SURGERY. *When this improvement occurs, your balance will improve, and you will then no longer be at risk for ulceration or amputation.*

There is hope for you. Visit Dellon.com or call +1 877-DELLON-1 (+1 877-335-5661) for more information.

3

Chapter Three
Joint Pain

"Joint pain might be due to a nerve injury."

Top Secret Meeting of the Joint Chiefs

The Chairman of the International Joint Chiefs was about to open the *top secret* meeting. Those able to attend the meeting in Switzerland, a neutral* country, are listed in Table 3-1.

Table 3-1. ATTENDANCE LIST OF JOINT CHIEFS MEETING; SWITZERLAND.

THE CHAIRMAN:
Eye Nose It-all, PhD (Anatomy), Italy

UPPER EXTREMITY:
Professor Doctor Shul der-Pien, MD, Holland
Doctor El-bow, Hurts-Alloviya, Spain
Barren Dr. Rist Ge Plotzen, Schmerze, Austria

LOWER EXTREMITY:
Le Docteur Knock Knies, MD, Tooloose, France
Sir Aincle Sprainagain, MD, Laxity, England

The Chairman introduced the subject, "Each of you Chiefs of Service is responsible for diagnosis and treatment of musculoskeletal pain in your unique, specialized, anatomic region. As you know, musculoskeletal pain demands that we assess the function of the ligaments, the bones, the cartilage, the muscles, and the very joints themselves. And we are excellent with this approach. Of course,," Doctor Nose It-all , continued, "there are always patients with real pain for whom our x-rays, our MRIS, and our traditional testing, say 'Normal.' The patient then may still come for surgery, for endoscopy, for joint replacement or fusion. We are usually excellent with this approach. But, *there are always the patients with persistent real pain.* And then, there is always referral to pain management. Yes, we are usually excellent with this approach too. But pain management represents our failure to understand the underlying source of the pain. It might be outside the musculoskeletal system!"

---

*Switzerland reportedly neither accepts nor denies the existence of nerves in joints but supports the right to investigate this matter further and bring it to the public's attention.

"Fellow Joint Chiefs, I now report to you the good news. Recently there was a report on the internet by Doctor Dellon that claimed joint pain might be due to a nerve injury! And I believe it too! We have all been missing something very important for our patients' pain relief. We must learn from Dr. Dellon's research. Please study his writings," he concluded. "Then we will meet again to discus this matter."

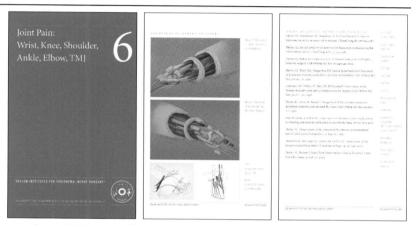

Figure 3-1. Brochure #6 from Dellon.com on Joint Denervation. This Brochure describes the scientific approach that I developed to treat joint pain and preserve joint function.

Partial Joint Denervation

"Doctor Dellon, I fell and hurts my wrist. The Orthopedic surgeon took x-rays. There were no fractures, but it really hurt. So he told me that I had badly sprained my wrist, and I had loose ligaments. He put me in a cast for three weeks so my torn ligaments could heal. But I still had pain. So he operated on me to tighten up my ligaments. That was two years ago! I still cannot move my wrist up or down without pain. Can you help me?" asked Valerie, a 26 year old woman. "It is my left hand and I am left handed. I have trouble writing even dressing my self," she added, frustrated.

"Yes, I can help you," I told her, "There are a group of small nerves that go to the wrist ligaments.. They now can be identified and removed."

"Will I still be able to move my wrist after that? Will I loose the feeling in my fingers after you remove those nerves," Valerie asked, worried.

"Your pain will be gone because I will remove just those nerves that were hurt when you fell. They only go to the ligaments of the joint. Those nerves do not control movement or sensation in the hand. They only send pain messages from the joint. The pain message will stop when I remove those damaged nerves. When your torn ligament healed, the nerves became stuck in the scar, forming a painful neuroma. My surgery will remove those damaged nerves," I explained.

"Doctor Dellon, why didn't the damaged nerves show up on the x-rays? Why didn't my Orthopedic surgeon tell me about these nerves?"

"Valerie," I answered her, "These nerves are too small to be seen by x-ray, and they are not even in any anatomy books the Orthopedic Surgeon, or even myself have studied. Valerie, beginning in 1977, I began to study the nerves to our joints. Fortunately, I have been able to learn about the location of the nerves to the wrist, then the knee, the shoulder, then the ankle and now the elbow. It is now possible to find these nerves and remove them, relieving pain in the joint and permitting the joint to more without pain."

"Doctor Dellon, how can you prove to me that you are right about why my wrist hurts?" Valerie asked, skeptical that nerves that were not in the anatomy books could really be the source of her pain.

"Valerie, here is the process we use. I will put a local anesthetic near the nerves I suspect are causing your pain. I will not put the local anesthetic into the joint itself. The you can see if your pain goes away, and if you can move your wrist better. If that happens, then we will have about a 90% chance of relieving your pain by removing the nerve that I block. Sometimes, for the wrist, two different nerves are injured, and I have to remove them both."

DOCTOR DELLON WON THE PLASTIC SURGERY EDUCATIONAL FOUNDATION SENIOR INVESTIGATOR RESEARCH AWARD IN 2005 FOR HIS CONCEPT OF PARTIAL JOINT DENERVATION.

"The nerve block," I continue, "is proof that if I remove the nerve it will not affect your ability to move your wrist and you will see that you do not loose sensation." (See Figure 3-2.)

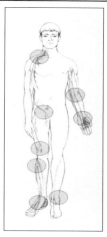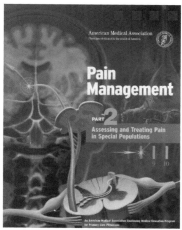

Figure 3-2. If a joint is injured in any part of the body, like the circled areas on the left, then the message from the nerves in that joint travel to the spinal cord, and then on to the brain, as illustrated on the right. The brain receives a message it interprets as joint pain. If a bone is not broken, but the nerve to the joint is stuck in the healed ligament of the joint, the brain understands that the joint hurts. If the joint has been removed and replaced, and the nerve to the original joint becomes stuck in scar around the joint replacement (the implant), then the brain receives a message of joint pain even in the absence of a joint.

Table 3-2. PRINCIPLES OF PARTIAL JOINT DENERVATION.

1. If your brain perceives pain in a joint, then that message is transmitted by a nerve

2. If the anatomy textbooks do not show nerves to a joint, then research can be done to identify those nerves. They do exist.

3. If the nerves to the joint can be found, then pain relief can be demonstrated by a local anesthetic nerve block.

4. If pain relief is possible by a nerve block of the nerve to the joint, then a surgical approach can be planned to remove that nerve.

5. If pain relief is possible by partial joint denervation, then joint function can be saved.

6. The above approach assumes that musculoskeletal structures have been restored, and the joint has structural stability.

The Wrist Joint

Valerie had a partial wrist denervation. In Figure 3-3, you can see her during our consultation and In Figure 3-4, you can see her improved wrist range of motion, which is now pain free.

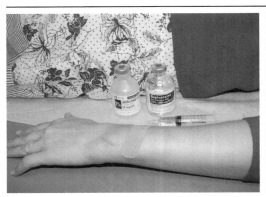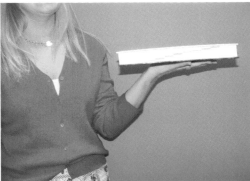

Figure 3-3. Two years after a wrist sprain and ligmanent reconstruction, Valerie still has severe left wrist pain. On the left, her wist is seen after local anesthetic block of the nerves to the wrist joint. On the right, 10 minutes later she is able to hold a heavy book against gravity without wrist pain. This successful wrist block indicates that she is an excellent candidate to have a partial wrist denervation procedure.

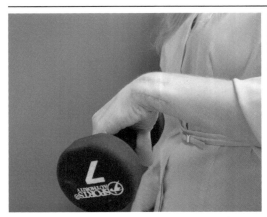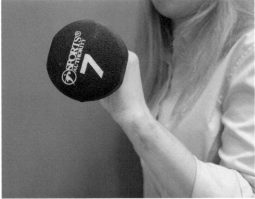

Figure 3-4. Valerie is shown 3 months after surgery flexing and extending her wrist without pain , holding a 7 pound weight. Her partial wrist denervation has been a success. Scars are from the original orthopedic surgery to stabilize her wrist. See Figure 3-5.

Wrist Assured of Pain Relief

Doctor Wilhelm, in Germany, in the 1960's began the modern era of wrist denervation. However, he believed that 5 incisions and 10 nerves needed to be removed. In 1979, I described the nerve to the back of the wrist joint and in 1984 the nerve to the front of the wrist joint. Today, total wrist denervation is still done for wrist pain, primarily in Europe. In papers in 1984 and 1985, I introduced the concept of just removing either the nerve to the front, or the nerve to the back of the wrist joint, as determined by nerve blocks. Today, both of these nerves can be removed through a single incision in the back of wrist. If wrist structure is strong, a long lasting result with improved function can be achieved. In Figure 3-3, the nerve block to the wrist with immediate relief of pain and improved function is demonstrated, and in Figure 3-4, the improved wrist function is demonstrated at 3 months. In Figure 3-5, a ten year result is illustrated.

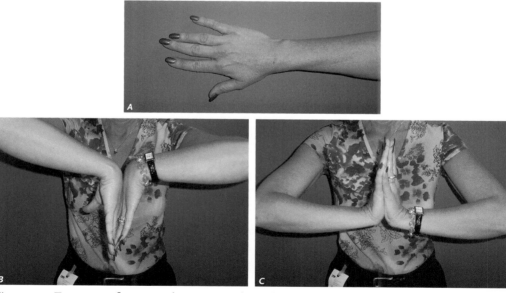

Figure 3-5. Ten years after wrist denervation through an incision over the back of the left wrist (A), there is a hardly noticeable scar. Wrist function is almost the same for the left and right wrists in flexion (B) and extension (C).

The concept of partial wrist denervation can also be applied to other joints in the hand. The bone behind the thumb, is a wrist bone called the trapezium. When there is severe arthritis, as in Figure 3-6, the trapezium is usually removed, in order to relieve pain and improve function.

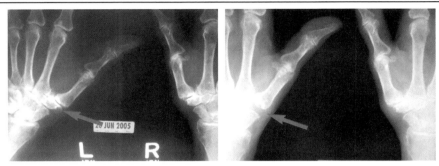

Figure 3-6. For severe arthritis of the wrist bone behind the thumb, called the trapezium, this bone is now usually completely removed and some form of spacer inserted. On the left x-ray, both the left and right trapezium have severe arthritis. In the right x-ray, note that the left trapezium (arrow) has been removed, and only a space remains on the x-ray.

In contrast consider Mindy's complaint. "Doctor Dellon, I am a piano player. When I play, I get horrible pains in the base of my thumbs near my wrist. I have seen two famous hand surgeons, who, based upon my x-rays (Figure 3-7) they both said I should have my trapezium removed, or my thumb joint fused. Dr. Dellon, if the Hand Surgeon does that, I cannot play the piano. Can you help me?"

"Yes, Mindy, I can help you. Let me examine your thumb," I said, and when I did examine her (Figure 3-7) I found that her pain was primarily in the front of the joint between the thumb and the trapezium.

"Mindy," I said, "if I remove just the bone spur and remove the nerve to the joint, in each hand, your pain will be relieved, and you will play the piano again."

Her result is noted in Figure 3-7, as she plays the piano.

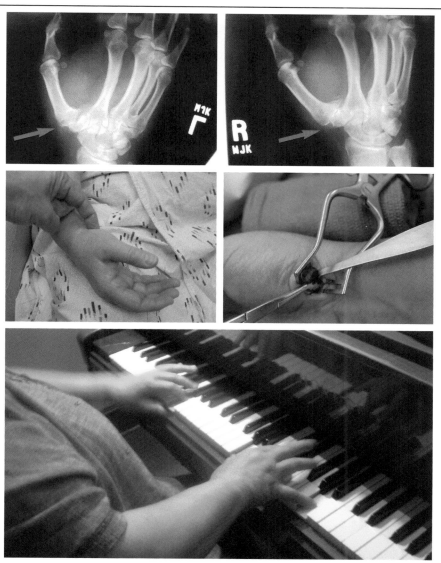

Figure 3-7. Top: X-rays of the left and right hand show severe trapezial arthritis. But examination of her hand (center left) demonstrated the pain to be only over a bone spur near the front, not the back, of the joint. Joint function could be preserved by removing the spur and denervating the thumb-trapezial joint. The intra-operative photo (center, right) demonstrates the spur removed (deep cavity) and the clamp holding the nerve to the joint. Bottom: After the same procedure on each hand, she is back playing piano.

The Knee Joint: A Great Pyrenees

We too often take pain-free walking for granted. If we develop knee pain from athletic injuries, or an accident, or from arthritis, then each step becomes painful and our daily activities are impaired. We can become disabled. From arthritis, this occurs so often that Orthopedic surgeons now replace 300,000 knee joints each year. The operation is successful, remarkably, about 97% of the time. But for those without such improvement, their remaining pain becomes intolerable, This exact situation occurs within the United States about 9,000 times per year. For some patients, the knee replacement surgery is so painful afterwards, and remains so painful, that they will not consider having the other arthritic knee replaced. This situation is illustrated in Figure 3-8.

As a Plastic Surgeon and Hand Surgeon, it was a surprise to me when Orthopedic surgeons began to send to me patients with knee pain. To my amazement, there were no nerves to the knee joint demonstrated in any anatomy book. The only nerve that was illustrated was a nerve to the skin that is located just below the knee cap (the infrapatellar branch of the saphenous nerve). This nerve clearly was in line to be cut by every long incision used in Orthopedic surgery in the front of the knee, and so that nerve was clearly not the problem. An example of this nerve, injured by an arthroscopic procedure in a teenage soccer player is given in Figure 3-9.

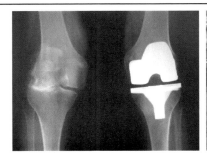 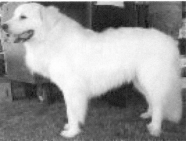

Figure 3-8. Left: Osteoarthritis is noted to be severe in the right knee. The left knee already has had a total knee arthroplasty, a knee joint replacement. When such a knee joint replacement still results in a painful knee, the patient just wishes to have a "Great Pyrenees." A Great Pyrenees dog is noted at right.

Patients who have a knee joint replaced and still have knee pain are a very unhappy group of patients. They have had a big operation. Usually they have had several operations before the knee replacement and yet still have pain. Rehabilitation was painful and are on narcotics and antidepressants (Figure 3-10).

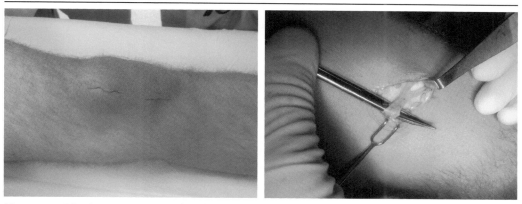

Figure 3-9. The known nerve to the skin below the knee cap (patella) is the infrapatellar branch of the saphenous nerve. Left: Ink marks an incision at the side of the patellar, and an arthroscopy portal (where the endoscope was put into the knee joint) below the patellar. The site below the patellar was painful. Right: At surgery, the infrapatellar branch is found and removed, leaving an area of numbness in place of the painful neuroma on the skin nerve.

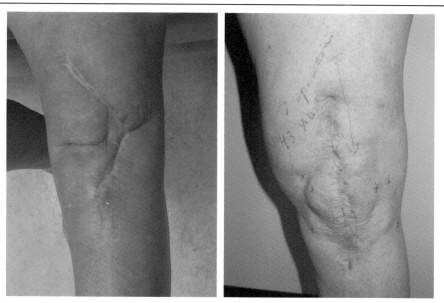

Figure 3-10. Examples of patients who still have pain after 18 (left) and 7 (right) previous knee operations. Each has had a total knee replacement and still has knee pain.

Removing the infrapatellar branch does NOT relieve knee *joint* pain. Therefore, in 1993, I began my research into the nerves to the knee joint.

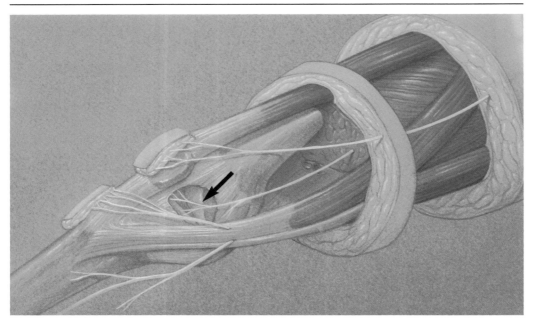

Figure 3-11A. Innervation of the human right knee joint. The medial (inside) view. Nerves to the skin and nerves to the knee joint are shown. Arrow points to the nerve to the medial aspect of the knee joint. This nerve is one of the main sources of medial knee join pain. With permission from Dellon.com.

This was published in 1994 (see reference in Figure 3-1, and Figure 3-11A and Figure 3-11B).

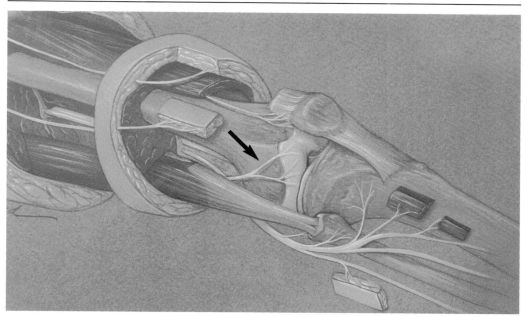

Figure 3-11B. Innervation of the human right knee joint. The lateral (outside) view. Nerves to the skin and nerves to the knee joint are shown. Arrow points to the nerve to the lateral aspect of the knee joint. This nerve is one of the main sources of lateral knee pain. With permission from Dellon.com.

Diagnosis of a Knee-Roma

The same approach used to develop my operations for partial wrist denervation was now applied to the knee joint. First, the nerves were identified through dissection of human cadavers, illustrated in Figure 3-11. Then patients who had a total knee replacement were evaluated with nerve blocks. Each patient must be at least 6 months after their knee replacement. If the patient had decrease in pain and could kneel and climb steps without pain after the nerve blocks, the presence of a neuroma of the nerve(s) to the knee joint was considered to be proven. At this point, the patient becomes a candidate for partial knee denervation surgery.

The relief of pain from partial knee denervation for patients who have had their knee replaced was so successful, it was incorporated into the leading book on knee surgery (Figure 3-13). This chapter contains the results of 344 patients with 90% good to excellent relief of knee pain. In most patients the nerve to the inside and the outside of the knee joint must be removed in addition to the infrapatellar branch of the saphenous nerve.

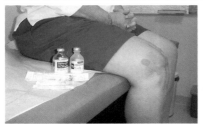
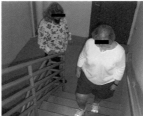
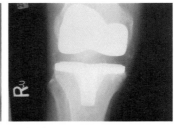

Figure 3-12. Nerve blocks are used to demonstrate that a nerve to the knee joint is the source of persistent pain after total knee replacement. Left: The anesthetics used for the block of just the nerves, not the knee joint. Center: Patient can climb stairs without pain after the nerve block, demonstrating improved function when the painful nerve is blocked. The patient is therefore an ideal candidate for a partial knee denervation procedure. Right: Demonstrates the excellent alignment of her knee replacement.

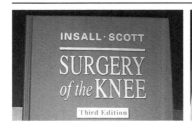
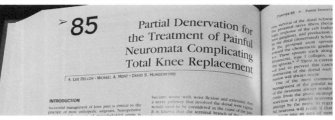

Figure 3-13. This 2000 edition of *Knee Surgery* contains Dellon's approach to partial knee denervation, and includes his first 344 patients that had this procedure done.

The surgery takes about an hour and a half. The surgery is done as an outpatient procedure. The patient walks immediately after the surgery, and usually knows the next day that the knee pain is finally gone. No rehabilitation is required. About one in twenty patients will need a second operation to remove a remaining painful nerve that was not detected at first.

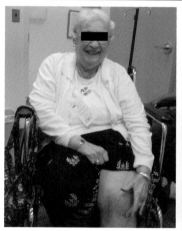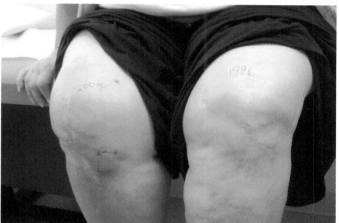

Figure 3-14. Examples of success after partial knee denervation in patients who have had pain. Left: This 82 year old woman has had 9 previous knee surgeries but still had disabling pain, essentially unable to walk. Here she is shown two weeks after her partial knee denervation procedure, smiling and ready to begin walking again. Right: A woman who had her left knee replaced in 1995, and had one of my first knee denervation procedures in 1996. Here she is seen in 2006, for her ten year follow-up. She came back because she now needs a partial knee denervation in her opposite leg which had a knee replacement one year ago.

At surgery, a small incision is made at each side of the knee, and the nerve to the joint, shown in Figure 11-10. A tourniquet is used so there is no bleeding, unlike the knee joint replacement procedure. Microsurgery is used to find the small nerves before they enter the scar around the knee implant. The knee implant is not exposed. After surgery, you know immediately that the knee joint pain is relieved. You walk immediately after the surgery. If the nerve to the skin has to be removed too, it is. This may make the skin more sensitive for a few weeks, and if this occurs walking in a heated swimming pool is then recommended. Otherwise there is no rehabilitation.

Knee Pain in the Athelete

Once I had proven that knee pain after knee joint replacement was due to nerves that innervated the knee joint, and that I could treat this knee pain by removing these nerves, then my challenge was to relieve knee pain in athletes. I assumed that these same small nerves would be torn in the injuries that tore the ligaments of the knee, and that removing these nerves would help also these young athletes.

Relief of knee pain with a local anesthetic block means that removing that nerve will relieve that pain; a successful block implies a 90% chance of success with knee joint denervation surgery.

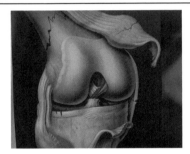

Figure 3-15. In the injured athlete, fractures to the knee cap (patella) or the bones about the knee, or rupture of the ligaments require musculoskeletal approaches to restore structural stability. But when this stability is restored, and there is still knee pain, the doctor must consider that this pain is coming from an injured nerve to the knee joint. (Image from a cover of the journal *Orthopedics*, in 2006.)

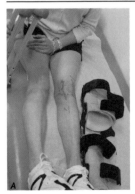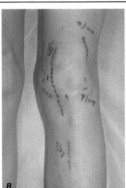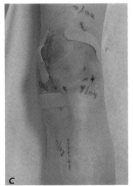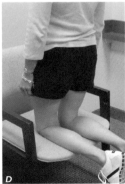

Figure 3-16. A young woman athlete is shown is A), disabled. Note her crutches and all her knee braces. B) Note the dates of each of the six surgeries she had within a two year time frame to treat her knee pain. c) Each band-aid is located at a site a nerve block. D) She has excellent relief of her knee pain, can climb steps and kneel down after the blocks, demonstrating that the remaining knee pain is due to small nerves torn in the injury.

The most common situation is to have a knee injury. Then to have an x-ray examination including an MRI. If a ligament is torn, it clearly needs to be reconstructed. If the MRI is normal and pain persists, or if the pain persists after the ligament is reconstructed, then pain due to a nerve injury must be considered. Knee pain of neurologic origin can be helped.

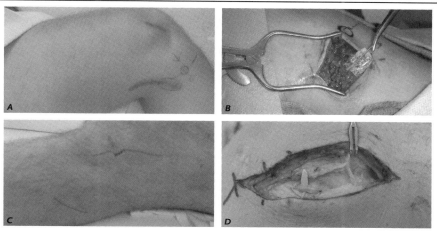

Figure 3-17. Two examples of male athletes with knee pain due to nerve injury. In A), this speed skater had had 8 years of knee pain. Shown is the site of his pain on the inside (medial) of the knee joint, where there is a scar from previous knee joint reconstruction. Neuroma pain site is marked by the circle and arrows. In B), a neuroma, held in the clamp in relationship to his site of pain at the medial knee. This nerve was removed and its end implanted into a nearby muscle. In c) a soccer player had lateral (outside) knee pain. The scar from the previous surgery on the joint is noted in blue. D) In surgery, the nerve injured and stuck in the scar is shown in relationship to the green marker. This nerve had to removed, and it was allowed to drop back behind the gate.

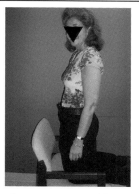

Figure 3-18. Ten years ago, this woman, then a younger athlete, suffered severe knee pain due to sports injuries. She had several musculoskeletal operations that restored strength and stability, but did not relieve her knee pain. Knee denervation surgery by Doctor Dellon returned her to a life where she can enjoy all the activity she still desires. Here she kneels, smiling, demonstrate her knee pain relief.

The Elbow Joint: Tennis Elbow and Golfer's Elbow

Tennis Elbow pain is on the outside of the elbow. Typically, the extension of the wrist required for the backswing puts a strain on the origin of the muscles on this (lateral) side of the elbow. The medical name for this is *lateral humeral epicondylitis,*

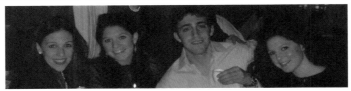

Figure 3-19. Like the mirror image twins pictured on either side of this young male professional lacrosse goalie, tennis elbow and golfer's elbow pain are quite similar, but, on opposite sides of the elbow their pain is transmitted by two different nerves. A future lawyer, seated on the far left, celebrates with the others that there is now a chance to treat elbow pain by treating the appropriate nerve that transmits the pain message to the brain.

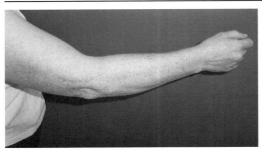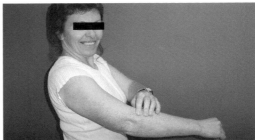

Figure 3-20. At two years after denervation of the right painful persistent tennis elbow, (left) the original painful tennis elbow scar is seen. Correction of that painful scar neuroma left the numb area noted by blue lines. Right: She smiles as she touches the previously painful area and extends her wrist now without tennis elbow pain.

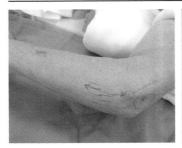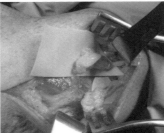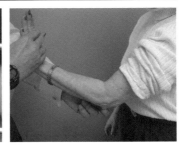

Figure 3-21. A woman who had previous surgery for her painful tennis elbow. Current pain site is noted by *, dashed blue line is the first surgical site scar. Dashed area is already numb due to nerve injury during previous surgery. Center: In surgery, the previously damaged nerves to skin and tennis elbow are shown on yellow background material prior to their removal. Right: Two years after Dr. Dellon's denervation surgery, she can extend wrist against resistance demonstrating relief of pain.

suggesting that inflammation from torn origins of the muscles from the elbow are the source of pain. While most people recover from Tennis Elbow with heat, anti-inflammatory medications, steroid injections, splinting and rest, about 10% due not. There are several Orthopedic surgical approaches for this problem which release the tendons, remove the inflamed tissue, and sometimes drill holes in the bone or even remove a piece of the bone. These approaches may fail to relieve pain, or the surgical approach may, itself injure a nerve to the skin on that side of the elbow. Alternatively, it is possible to remove the small nerves that carry the pain message from the covering of the lateral humeral epicondyle, the bone from which these muscles arise, and thereby stop the pain message to the brain.

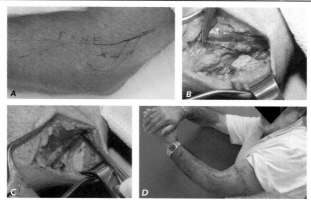

Figure 3-22. A man with disabling tennis elbow pain who has had no previous surgery. A: Before surgery, the * notes the site of his pain. The other lines are the proposed location of the nerves to the site of the pain, the lateral humeral epicondyle (LHE) and the nerve to the skin, the posterior cutaneous nerve of the forearm (PCNF). In B, in surgery, the nerve to the LHE is seen on the blue background material, and the PCNF is held in the clamp. These two nerves join to become one nerve, which is then, in C turned and implanted into the triceps muscle to prevent them from growing back and causing pain again. D: Just one day after surgery, he smiles as his pain is gone and he can extend his wrist against resistance without pain. He will be able to use his hand immediately and by three weeks do as he wishes with his hand and elbow. Typically, no rehabilitation is required.

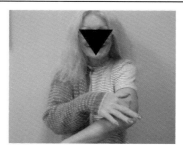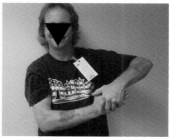

Figure 3-23. More people relieved of tennis elbow pain by denervation surgery.

Golfer's Elbow or Throwers Elbow are both conditions in which the same pain discussed above for Tennis Elbow occurs on the inside of the elbow. This pain is caused when the wrist is pulled or flexed, instead of extended. This condition is common in baseball pitchers. Again, the problem is most often successfully treated without surgery, but, again , there are Orthopedic surgical procedures that alter the origin of the muscles that arise from the medial humeral epicondyle (MHE), the inside of the elbow bone. The good news is that in 2006, Doctor Dellon published a paper related to the nerve that carries the pain message from this bone and its muscles.* The nerve had not been described before.

The really good news is that now this medial elbow pain can be relieved by removing this nerve. In addition to sports injuries, the medial elbow pain

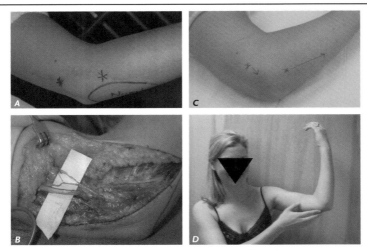

Figure 3-24. Two patients who have had previous surgery for ulnar nerve entrapment at the elbow, which is called cubital tunnel syndrome and who still have not only ulnar nerve entrapment but also elbow pain. In A, note the long incision from the first ulnar nerve transposition surgery. The two * indicates the site of the bone pain at the elbow and the site of the painful neuroma to the skin. B: In surgery, the small nerves to the elbow are noted, and will be removed. (Photos courtesy of Chistopher T.Maloney, Jr., MD, Tucson, Dellon Institute for Peripheral Nerve Surgery). In c the previous incision is noted from the earlier two ulnar nerve surgeries. Again the two * indicates the site of the bone pain at the elbow and the site of the painful neuroma to the skin. In D the patient is shown three months after the nerves have been removed. She can touch the previously painful area now without pain , evidenced by her smile.

*Dellon AL, Ducic I, DeJesus RA: Innervation of the Medial Humeral Epicondyle: Implications for Medial Epicondylar Pain, J Hand Surg, 31B:331-333, 2006.

can be a complication of elbow surgery to decompress the ulnar nerve. This nerve becomes compressed in the *cubital tunnel.* Surgery to decompress the ulnar nerve in the cubital tunnel can create a neuroma of the nerve to the skin and the nerve to the bone. If a patient has pain when the ulnar nerve surgery scar is touched and the pain goes to the little finger, the ulnar nerve is still compressed. If the pain goes to the elbow or forearm skin, there is a neuroma of the medial antebrachial cutaneous nerve. But if the pain is felt to be in the elbow itself, then the same nerve that causes the pain of Golfer's elbow and thrower's elbow is the source of this elbow pain.

Elbow pain, that is not due to bone fragments in the joint, is most likely due to injury to the nerves to the elbow joint. These painful nerves can be removed. Partial elbow denervation offers hope for elbow pain.

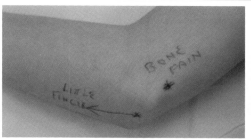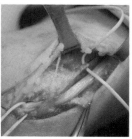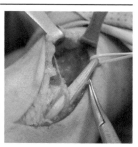

Figure 3-25. Twelve year old girl who injured her right elbow falling during soccer. There were no fractures but she had persistent elbow pain and numbness in her little and ring fingers. Left: One year after her fall she had both bone pain localized at the * and evidence of ulnar nerve compression in the cubital tunnel. Center: In surgery, the compressed ulnar nerve is encircled with a blue rubber band, while the nerve to the medial humeral epicondyle lies over the loose blue rubber band. This is the nerve that also causes Golfer's and Thrower's Elbow pain. Right: This nerve has been removed and its end placed into the triceps muscle in the dark tunnel beneath the retractors.

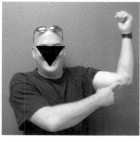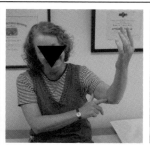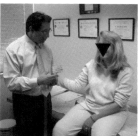

Figure 3-26. Three more patients who have had relief of their medial elbow pain by denervation of the medial humeral epicondyle. In the right example, the woman can flex her wrist against resistance, which is the movement that causes Golfer's Elbow pain.

Shoulder Joint: Bursa, Rotator Cuff, or Nerve?

Do you have shoulder pain? Did you injure and tear your rotator cuff? Did you have your rotator cuff repaired and still have shoulder pain? PERSISTENT SHOULDER PAIN CONTINUES IN 20% OF PEOPLE AFTER ROTATOR CUFF REPAIR!

Do you have shoulder pain? Did you have arthritis in your shoulder due to aging, an old fracture, or subacromial bursitis? PERSISTENT SHOULDER

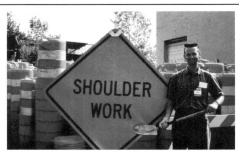

Figure 3-27. Doctor Oskar Aszmann, in 1995, when he was doing the basic anatomy dissections with me to demonstrate the existence and pattern of the nerves to the shoulder joint. This research was critical to my approach to shoulder denervation to relieve joint pain. Note the microsurgical dissecting tools he is using. He is now Associate Professor of Plastic Surgery at the University of Vienna, in Austria, and a leading nerve researcher.

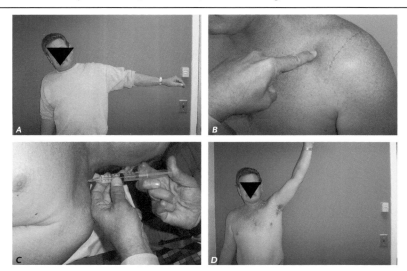

Figure 3-28. A: This man has had a rotator cuff repair but still has left shoulder pain and cannot lift the left arm higher than shown here without pain. Note position of white box on the blue wall as a marker of this height. B: First step is to prove that the shoulder pain is coming from a nerve. This is done with a local anesthetic as shown in C. D: Fifteen minutes after the block, his pain is gone, and he can lift his left arm. Note position of the white box as a marker. This means that he should get a great response from a left partial shoulder denervation. Just the nerve to the front of the joint is removed at surgery.

PAIN CONTINUES IN 20% OF PEOPLE AFTER SUBACROMIAL PLASTY, the operation for shoulder joint inflammation.

Do you have shoulder pain? Have you had to have your shoulder joint replaced due to arthritis after a fracture, or rheumatoid arthritis? Well, PERSISENT SHOULDER PAIN EVEN CAN CONTINUE AFTER A SHOULDER JOINT REPLACEMENT.

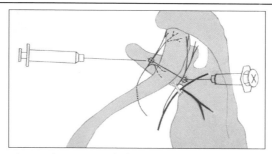

Figure 3-29. This figure shows the approach for the nerve block to the front of the shoulder joint of the nerve identified through our anatomic research. The nerve is a sensory branch from the motor nerve to the pectoralis muscle.

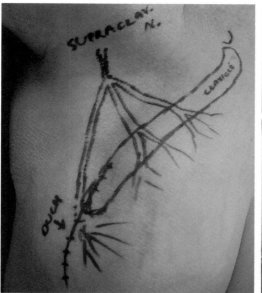
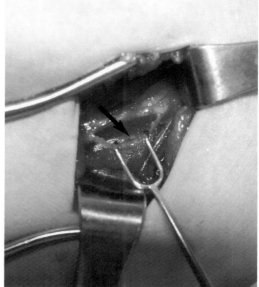

Figure 3-30. Left: The surgery. With the patient under general anesthesia, a drawing was made to show the colar bone (clavicle). The blue hatched line is the scar from previous orthopedic shoulder surgery. The supraclavicular nerve is shown (arrow). This nerve is only for the skin sensation and does not give shoulder pain. Care is taken to save this nerve when only a shoulder denervation is done. Right: A small incision is made below the clavicle, near the shoulder, the pectoralis muscle is spread apart, and the small nerve to the shoulder capsule is indentified. This nerve is then removed to relieve the shoulder pain.

The surgery is done with the patient asleep under general anesthesia. An incision is made below the colar bone, the chest muscle (pectoralis) is spread apart to find the small nerve to the front of the shoulder joint. This nerve is removed. You can move your arm and use your hand immediately after the operation. This shoulder denervation assumes that the Orthopedic surgery has reconstructed the shoulder ligaments and the muscles have sufficient strength, and that there are no scars limited joint mobility. Then you can raise your arm immediately following the surgery.

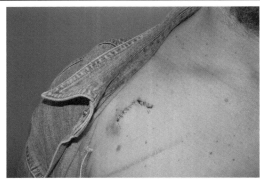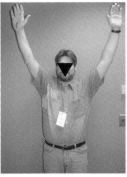

Figure 3-31. Immediately following the shoulder denervation, you can begin to use your shoulder. Left: The scar for the shoulder denervatrion is shown 5 days after the surgery. Right: On that same day, the right shoulder can be raised as high as the left without pain. Shoulder denervation surgery assumes that shoulder joint itself is strong and that the shoulder pain is coming from the nerve, which was injured originally.

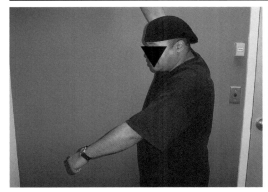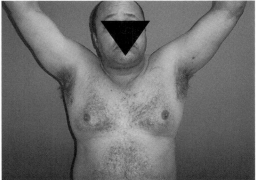

Figure 3-32. This man had two shoulder arthroscopies but remained with pain. Left: Note the left arm could not be lifted more than this without shoulder pain. After the nerve block he had less pain and improved his shoulder range of motion. This meant that he would be a good candidate for shoulder denervation. Right: One month after surgery, he can lift his left shoulder without pain.

When the skin is hypersensitive or painful in addition to the shoulder joint being painful, then the supraclavicular nerve branch to the original shoulder surgery scar can be removed. This nerve is found at the shoulder, traced into the neck, where it originated, and removed. This leaves numbness in the previously painful shoulder skin area, but the skin pain is gone. An example of this type of surgery is illustrated in Figure 3-33.

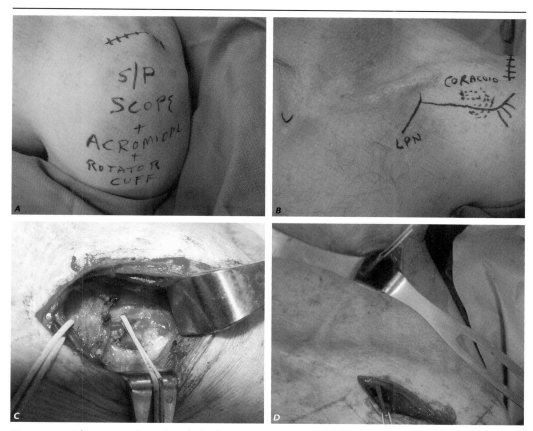

Figure 3-33. The patient has already had, as noted in A, a shoulder arthroscopy, an acromioplasty and a rotator cuff repair but still has disabling shoulder pain, and has hypersensitive skin. B: the front view indicates the location of the nerve to the pectoralis muscle, the lateral pectoral nerve (LPN), whose motor function is preserved, and the branch that we remove going towards the shoulder joint. This branch crosses the bone called the coracoid, which is why the nerve block is done in that location. In surgery, C the two blue rubber bands are each around a nerve. The larger nerve to the left is the one that goes to the painful skin, and arises in the neck, and the smaller one goes to the shoulder joint and will be removed first. D: The nerve to the skin is shown in the incision near the shoulder, and its origin in the neck is not shown. This nerve will be removed too, so that instead of painful shoulder skin, there will be an area of numbness. After this surgery, both the skin pain and the shoulder joint pain will be gone.

Shoulder Joint Replacement Surgery

If shoulder pain persists even after replacement of the shoulder joint, a consideration should be that the pain is coming from a nerve to the

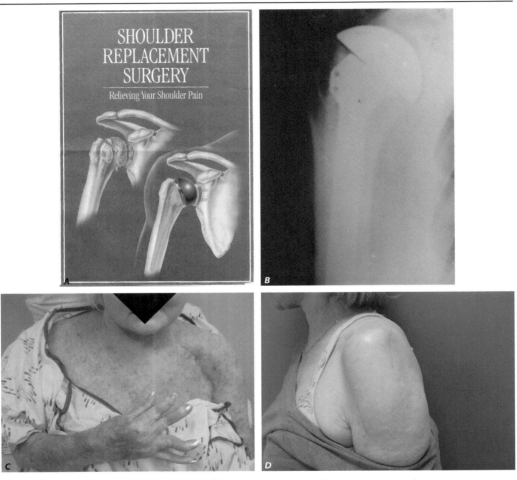

Figure 3-34. A: Cover of the journal Orthopedics featured shoulder joint replacement. B: An x-ray of a new shoulder joint in place. C and D: Patients whose shoulder joints have been replaced, but they still have shoulder pain. The * on the woman's shoulder in c) shows the site of persistent pain. This can be helped by the shoulder denervation surgery.

shoulder joint that is stuck in scar around the new shoulder joint implant. If that is true, then there is hope that the pain can be relieved by a joint denervation.

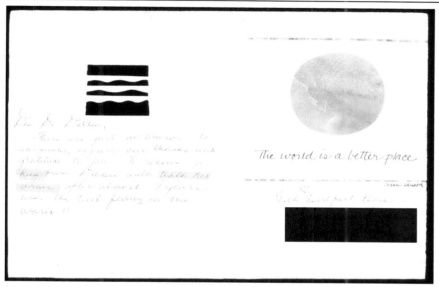

Figure 3-35. I received this card in 1997. It was from one of my first partial shoulder joint denervation patients. The card reads, "Dear Dr. Dellon, There are just no words to adequately express our thanks and gratitude to you. To receive a hug from Debbie with both her arms after almost 7 years was the best feeling in the world."

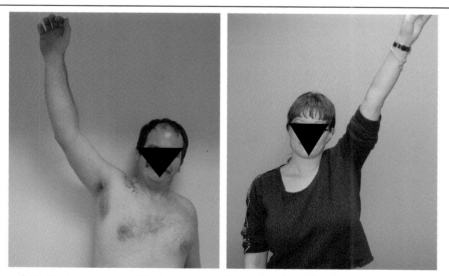

Figure 3-36. Patients wave good by to us as we leave the shoulder denervation section of this chapter. Each of them is waving to us with a hand that could not be lifted above the shoulder level due to shoulder pain. Each has had a shoulder joint partial denervation procedure.

The Ankle Joint

If you have ever sprained your ankle, you know the intense immediate excruciating pain you feel as the ligaments that hold the ankle bones together rips apart. With ice, anti-inflammatory medication, and some form of a splint, pain usually subsides quickly. Immobilization, keeping the bones and ligaments from moving, helps healing, but it also stops the nerves within the ligaments of the ankle joint to stop sending pain signals.

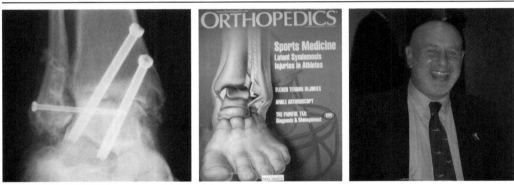

Figure 3-37. Left: "Screwed" fixing a fractured ankle. Center: Torn ligaments on journal cover; no nerves are illustrated. Right: Why is this man smiling? He knows pain can be relieved by getting rid of something. "It is OK to lose your nerve. Lose it and use it" he says.

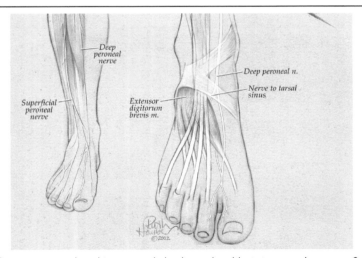

Figure 3-38. The nerves to the skin around the lateral ankle joint are the superficial peroneal nerve shown in yellow, and the sural nerve, not shown, behind the lateral ankle bone. The deep peroneal nerve, yellow, crosses the top of the ankle and sends branches to the sinus tarsi region. This illustration is from the Dellon.com website.

"Wait, what did you say? There are nerves sending pain signals from the ankle joint?" a shrill voice from medical knowledge screams out. "No way. The anatomy books do not show any nerves to the ankle joint," the hysterical, historical voice concludes its objections.

Really good news! There are nerves to the ankle joint. These nerves can be blocked with local anesthetic. If pain is relieved by a nerve block, these nerves can be removed and your pain can be relieved.

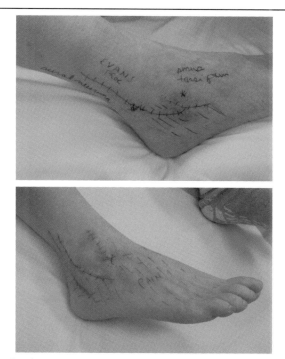

Figure 3-39. Two ankles that have required surgery for their fracture/dislocations. The surgical scars are outlined with blue hatched lines. Areas of painful skin are shown outlined by the blue ink dashes. Top: The location of the disabling sinus tarsi pain is shown by the * and the words "sinus tarsi." The second * is located over the words "sural neuroma" and is the site where the sural nerve was injured and stuck in the surgical approach for the Evans procedure, a procedure used to tighten the loose lateral ankle ligaments. Bottom: There have been three operations already on this painful ankle. The * is located over the sinus tarsi. The blue ink dashes indicate painful skin due to both the sural nerve and the superficial peroneal nerve. The good news is that even with this much previous surgery and long lasting pain, the nerve to the sinus tarsi, the deep peroneal nerve, can be removed, relieving the ankle joint pain. The nerves to the skin, the sural nerve and the superficial peroneal nerves also can be removed, leaving the skin area numb. The end of the nerve is implanted in a muscle above the ankle, so that wearing a shoe no longer causes pain when the skin is touched.

When the fracture or dislocation or bad sprain occurs on the outside of the ankle, the most common place for it to occur, ligaments that surround a space called the *Sinus Tarsi* get torn. In the approach to correct the fracture and the ligaments, the Foot and Ankle surgeon may need to tighten or reconstruct the ligaments in addition to corrected the fractures. This creates the possibility for lateral ankle pain to be due to injuries (neuromas) of the nerves to the skin as well as nerves to the joints. Both sources of nerve pain must be corrected to relieve pain on the lateral aspect of the ankle. In Chapter 1, the concepts related to removing the painful nerve and implanting it into a muscle were discussed and illustrated.

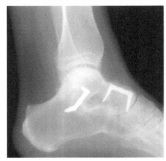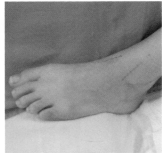

Figure 3-40. This woman injured her left ankle 7 years ago. She has already had three ankle surgeries. The last one, shown (left) demonstrates the metal clips where she had had her ankle fused. Her ankle still hurts despite its fusion. Right: The previous surgical scars created painful skin that she would not even let the bed sheets touch. She used a cane or crutches despite having an ankle fusion. She had a denervation of her sinus tarsai (removal of the deep peroneal nerve). She also had removal the superficial peroneal nerve to remove the source of pain to the skin. Immediately after surgery, she could touch the skin and press on the sinus tarsi region without the previous pain. Finally, she can walk without ankle pain.

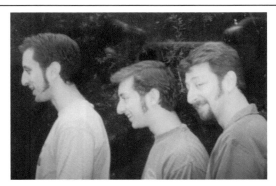

Figure 3-41. "Hair" today, Gone tomorrow. And so it can be for Nerve Pain. "Here" today, and Gone tomorrow. Partial Joint Denervation makes this possible. "It is OK to lose your nerve," as long as the correct nerve is chosen to lose.

Here we focus on the pain in the lateral ankle joint, and the sinus tarsi region.

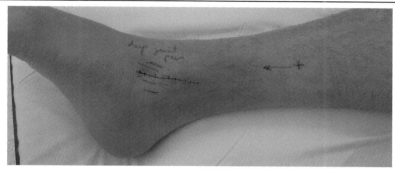

Figure 3-42. The inside of the ankle, the medial ankle, can hurt too. This man had a fracture of the ankle requiring an incision, hatched blue line, over the medial mallelous. He now has painful skin in this region and deep medial ankle pain. This type of pain can be due to the branches of the saphenous nerve. The * is where tapping on the saphenous nerve causes pain to go into the painful skin and the ankle. A nerve block in this location will relieve the pain, permitting walking without ankle pain, and touching the numb skin.

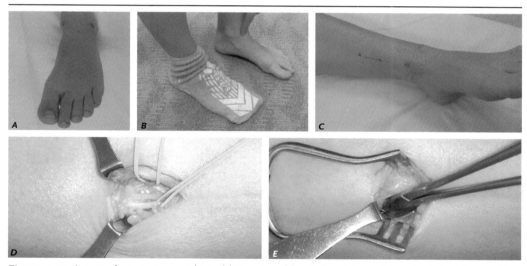

Figure 3-43. A marathon runner and triathlete injured her left ankle, and has had disabling ankle pain for four years. A: The two ink marks are the site of her first operation, and arthroscopic ankle surgery which left her with worse pain, both on the inside (medial) and outside (lateral) aspect of her ankle. The S-shaped scar across the front of her ankle is from a neurosurgical attempt to remove scar tissue from her superficial peroneal nerve. This did not help her either. B: She points to the site of her medial ankle pain. C: the * indicates the site where a nerve block of the saphenous nerve relieved the medial ankle pain. The blue dash marks are where she has scar directly at the medial ankle arthroscope portal. D: The saphenous nerve branches are encircled by the blue rubber bands. The saphenous vein is noted between them. These two nerve branches are removed and, in E the nerve ends are implanted into the underlying muscle. Her functional results are demonstrated in Figure 3-44. She has had great pain relief.

There are many individual joints related to the ankle, and there are also joints between the ankle bones and the toes bones. It is critical to be sure there are no remaining bone fragments in these joints before doing the denervation procedures. As note above, in some patients, an injured nerve to the skin of the foot must also be removed to relieve the foot and ankle pain in addition to the partial ankle joint denervation procedures.

PRINCIPLES OF PARTIAL JOINT DENERVATION:

There are nerves to the joints, these nerves can be the source of pain, these nerves can be removed, nerve blocks determine which nerves to remove.

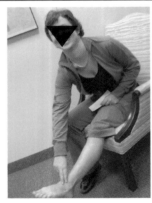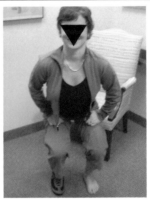

Figure 3-44. The marathon runner and triathlete, whose left ankle pain problem is shown in Figure 3-43, first had an operation to help the lateral side of her ankle, to treat her sinus tarsi pain problem. She touches the lateral aspect of her foot (left), where removal of the deep peroneal nerve helped her lateral ankle pain. That surgery was six months ago. Right. She is just one day after the surgery for her medial ankle pain. The saphenous nerve was removed, as described in Figure 3-43. Her she is shown squatting down with full ankle flexion without pain. "Doctor Dellon," she said, "Before surgery I could not do squat without pain. Now I can squat without any pain. Thank you Doctor Dellon."

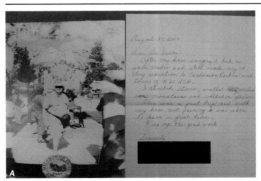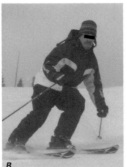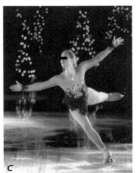

Figure 3-45. Improved function and enjoyment of life after partial joint denervation.
A: After knee denervation, B and C after ankle denervation.

Pain Solutions Summary

Joint pain must first be considered to be due to a problem related to the ligaments, bones, cartilage that make up the structure and function of a joint. However, it must never be forgotten that the pain experienced is transmitted from these structures to the brain by a peripheral nerve. *When joint pain continues after all aspects of the musculoskeletal system have been treated, then the remaining source of joint pain must be considered to come from an injured nerve.*

Although traditional textbooks do not document the presence of nerves in joints, Doctor Dellon's research has documented the presence of nerves in joints. Surgeons trained in microneurosurgery can identify these nerves, and these nerves can be removed by appropriately designed surgical procedures. *The Dellon partial joint denervation procedure is demonstrated to be successful for the shoulder, elbow, wrist, knee, and ankle joints. Partial joint denervation can relieve pain and preserve joint function.*

There is hope for you.

Visit Dellon.com or call +1 877-DELLON-1 (+1 877-335-5661).

4

Chapter Four
Groin Pain

"There is a *demon* attached to my pubic bone!"

When Can I Have Sex Again?

Joan (not her real name) was an airline stewardess. She was born in the Caribbean. She was lively, and a real fun person to be with. She enjoyed intimate relationships. That was before she had her hernia repair!

Joan now lives in Boston. She is 31 years old. She thinks she may have gotten her hernia pushing those heavy beverage and food carts in the airplanes. She had her left inguinal (groin) hernia repaired in March of 2001. She awoke with horrible stabbing pain in her groin area. The pain never went away.

Her doctor, an experienced general surgeon, told her the surgery had no complications, and that the hernia was fixed. The incision was healing well. The piece of plastic mesh put into the hernia site to give it strength was not the source of her pain, he reassured her. He renewed her oxycodone (her narcotic pain medication).

Three weeks after the surgery, when the surgical pain should have been gone, the surgeon continued her pain medicine. He told Joan her left groin area might hurt a little while longer and to come back in 2 more months. He renewed her oxycodone. Joan was not able to return to work at the airline due to pain.

Three months after the surgery, when Joan still complained of pain in her pubic area and in the inside of her left thigh, her surgeon told her he still did not know why she was having pain. Joan showed him the spot that set off the pain. She could put her left index finger directly on the spot near her incision that set off the pain. He sent her for a special x-ray study, an MRI, of her pelvis. This showed that the hernia was fixed, and there were no new problems that could cause this pain. He told Joan she could work, if she wanted to work, and she should come back in three more months. He discontinued her oxycodone and told her to take Advil™, so she would not become addicted to the drugs.

Joan could not bend over without the pain. She could not wear a dress or pants with a tight top. Due to the pain in her groin, she was uncomfortable having intimate relationships. And stopped having them. She asked for a referral to a Pain Management doctor.

Joan finally came to be cared for by Dr. J (not his real name), a very successful Pain Management doctor in Boston. She continued trying different medications from the Pain Management doctor. He was very sympathetic. He tried giving her nerve blocks, and these actually relieved the pain, but only for a few hours. This proved that pain was coming from an injured nerve.

When the non-narcotic pain medications did not help her, she resumed taking narcotics, the type that had long lasting effects, throughout the day. Her income stopped. In time she had to leave her apartment and move in with relatives. She no longer had intimate relationships.

Joan became addicted to narcotics. She saw none of her old friends.

Three years after her hernia surgery, Dr. J. referred her to me. Dr. J. knew of my special interest, Peripheral Nerve Surgery, because he had a patient whom I had helped greatly the previous year. That patient was unable to move his toes, was reduced to a wheel chair from a very active life, and was dependent upon all forms of pain medication every day. That patient came to see me in Baltimore, where I am Director of the Dellon Institutes for Peripheral Nerve Surgery®. As a Plastic Surgeon, I have been trained to solve difficult, and often unique, problems. I devised a plan to correct the injured nerves that proved to be successful for Dr. J's patient with leg pain, and so now Dr J. felt comfortable to refer Joan to me.

Joan, accompanied by three family members, traveled to Baltimore to see me. On the wall in my office is an illustration of the different nerves that can cause groin pain. Each nerve pain territory is shown in a different color.

Joan pointed to the area of the chart **(see Figure 4-1)** that matched her pain. She then showed me the area that triggered her pain. **When she would lie down , and when she would sit up, the pain came on intensely.**

"I can help you with this Joan," I said. "I can fix this problem."

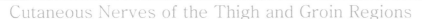

Cutaneous Nerves of the Thigh and Groin Regions

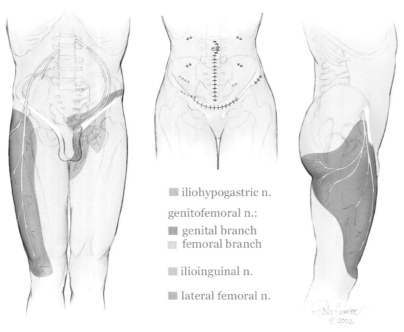

iliohypogastric n.

genitofemoral n.:
■ genital branch
femoral branch

■ ilioinguinal n.

■ lateral femoral n.

Figure 4-1. Groin Pain of Neural Origin. Each color represents the skin region innervated by the nerve represented by the same color. The scars represent typical operations, listed in Table 4-1. The location of the scar is in the same color as the nerve that is usually injured in that location. If your pain is related to these areas, then your pain is of neural origin. (with permission from http://ww.dellon.com)

Her pain was due to an injury of the ilioinguinal nerve, a nerve that travels in the same area in which the hernia was repaired. This is the nerve that is the usual cause of pain after hernia repair, although there are four different nerves to consider. The nerve can become trapped in the sutures used for the hernia repair or become trapped in the mesh. When Joan would sit up or lie down, the nerve would be pulled by the muscles against the scar, setting off the pain. The temporary relief she obtained with the nerve block proved this to be true.

I explained that the surgery would take one hour, and would be done under general anesthetic. Joan would be an outpatient and could walk immediately after the surgery.

Joan asked the critical questions that concerned her: How soon would it be till she knew she was better? How long would it take her to be able to work again? How long would it be before she could have sexual intercourse again? I told her there were no guarantees of success, but there was a 90% chance she could resume her previous activities, and that Doctor J. would work with her then to reduce her dependence on drugs.

Joan consulted with her family. She decided to have the surgery.

I operated on Joan three weeks later. It was April of 2005. Joan had been in pain for more than four years.

At surgery, I made a new incision in front of her left hip bone. I found the ilioinguinal nerve, and removed it. There was no need to remove the mesh or disrupt the original hernia repair.

Joan awoke in the recovery room. When her mind began to let her appreciate her condition, she reached down and touched the trigger spot. There was no pain. But she vaguely remembered that I had told her I would put a local anesthetic into the skin so she would awake without pain from the incision itself. Then she pressed down really hard. There was no pain! Joan suddenly sat up on the stretcher in the recovery room. There was no pain! Her nurse saw her sit up, and, fearing some medical emergency, came quickly to her side. Joan whispered something to the nurse. I had just come back into the recovery room to check on Joan. The nurse looked up in surprise, as Joan, with a wide-eyed stare, and a smile, repeated her question loudly:

"When can I have sex again?"

Dave's Groin Pain

Dave L. (not his real name) works in Hollywood. He is a writer and a director. He does his homework. When his right groin pain was said to be due to an inguinal hernia, he did his research. He chose a general surgeon to do the hernia repair who used the latest approach. This approach did not make an incision, but relied upon small "punctures" made through the abdomen, and through these holes (endoscopic sites) corrected the hernia by placing a piece of plastic mesh into the weak abdominal wall. The mesh is held in place by small "tacks." The surgeon had done this procedure many times without problems. In fact, he was known to have done this on many famous Hollywood "stars." So Dave signed up to have his hernia fixed by this experienced surgeon using an endoscopic mesh technique.

In 1996, Dave went to sleep with his dull, aching, right groin, hernia pain. He had puncture wounds placed near his belly button and in his right groin to permit the hernia repair with the mesh and the tacks. Although his surgeon was to tell him later that the surgery went "perfectly and without complications," Dave says he awoke with *"a demon attached to my pubic bone."* His pain never stopped.

Dave, like Joan mentioned earlier in this chapter, went through the ritual of wound healing pain, normal post-operative pain, prolonged surgical pain. He went through the sequence of pain medication to chronic pain medication. He went to other surgeons for second and then third, and then fourth opinions. He went to the famous West Coast Universities of Stanford and UCLA, seeking answers from neurologists, radiologists, surgeons, and finally pain management doctors. Dave became depressed, disillusioned with the medical profession, and a typical chronic pain patient.

Dave was told that his pain was due to a nerve injury, but that he should not have that nerve cut.

Dave bravely showed his x-ray to anyone who would look and listen (see Figure 4-2 for a similar x-ray.). The x-ray that showed the metal tacks, he was told, did not mean that any of those tacks was the source of his pain, even though one of those tacks was exactly where he felt the "demon" was gnawing on his pubic bone.

Dave could no longer do creative writing due to his pain, and he dropped off the Hollywood radar screen. Dave could no longer maintain the loving relationship with his wife due to his chronic pain. His personality changed.

He no longer derived pleasure playing with his young son. His wife went back to work as a lawyer to provide an income for their family.

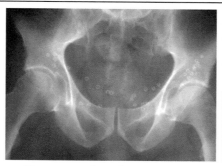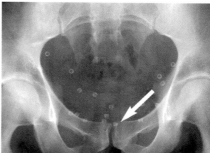

Figure 4-2. X-ray examples of patients who each had endoscopic bilateral hernia repair using plastic mesh and metal tacks to hold the mesh. These tacks may painfully impinge a nerve against a bone (arrow), or encircle the nerve beneath the skin.

Dave grew a beard, and began to search the internet looking for the help that he prayed was out there, somewhere. The internet located a scientific paper written by A. Lee Dellon, MD, a Plastic Surgeon in Baltimore. Doctor Dellon had begun to identify the relationships between the nerves that innervate the groin, and groin pain of neural origin. Dave e-mailed me for help.

I asked Dave by e-mail if he could point to an area that set off the pain He replied "yes, but no one is willing to operate on me again to remove a nerve or a metal tack."

I replied by e-mail "There is hope for you. I can help you." I asked Dave to come to Baltimore to see me. He said he was in too much pain to fly I was scheduled to lecture at a University in San Francisco shortly thereafter, and asked Dave if he though he could make the trip from LA to San Francisco. Dave came up from LA to see me. I listened to his story, reviewed the x-ray, and examined him.

"I can help you Dave," I said. "I want to propose a special approach to solve this problem for you. There are so many tacks and I want to be sure to remove the right one."

"What approach will you use," Dave asked?

I explained that the surgery would begin with Dave under twilight sleep, while I used a local anesthetic to make the skin numb for the incision. Then the anesthesiologist would wake him up sufficiently so that he would know I was touching him inside the wound. Dave would then tell me his pain level as I explored the depths of the wound to find the tack. When I had touched the exact trigger spot for his pain he would tell me. Then the anesthesiologist would put him completely to sleep and I would remove the tack in that location. The intravenous medications would remove the memory of most of this experience for him. Dave agreed to the plan, and flew to Baltimore.

The surgery was in October of 1999. Dave had been in pain for three years. Dave awoke from surgery and smiled. He knew immediately. "The demon is gone." He went back to the West Coast.

In three months he was off his narcotic medications, and his head and creative powers returned. He began writing again for a major studio. He regained his strength. He wrote to me.

"My wife and I are like back when we were in college, having enjoyable sex regularly."

Later that year, Dave sent me, a Holiday Card, with a photo of himself, his wife, and his son, wearing their ski gear. They had gone to Lake Tahoe, and were standing on the mountain on the California trail, with views of both California and Nevada. Dave wrote on the card,

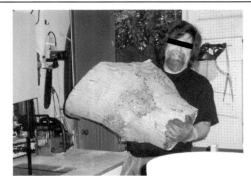

Figure 4-3. Smiling Dave, lifting a log in his workshop, 6 years after Dellon procedure for groin pain.

"My family and I are on the top of the world again, thanks to you."

In 2005, Dave and I connected again by e-mail. He sent me a picture of himself, carrying a large tree trunk in his wood working shop at home. He could lift, use power tools, and give in fully to his creative spirit. A wide smile shown though his beard. Still free of groin pain 6 years and counting.

Hernia Surgery and Groin Pain Statistics

It has been estimated that there are 700,000 hernia repairs done each year in the United States. Scientific outcome studies in 2001 and 2003 found that about 50% of patients after hernia repair have some degree of prolonged pain, and that 25% have pain for more than one year.* One in eight patients have functionally disabling pain more than one year after hernia repair.**

What Types of Surgery can cause Groin Pain?

The types of surgery that may result in groin pain are given in Table 4-1. Any incision in the lower abdomen or upper thigh may injure a nerve and result in groin pain.

Table 4-1.

Types of Operations that can Cause Groin Pain due to Nerve Injury:

Abdominoplasty	Hysterectomy
Angioplasty	Hernia Repair
Breast Reconstruction	Femoral
(tram flap)	Inguinal (with or without mesh)
Cardiac Catheterization	Ventral Abdominal Wall
Femoral Artery Surgery	Ileostomy/Colostomy
Gastric By-Pass	Orchiectomy

*Bay-Nielsen, Annals of Surgery, 233:1-7, 2001, and Rutkow, Surgical Clinics of North America, 73:413-426, 2003.

**Dellon, A.L., Invited Discussion of Pain Complications after Hernia Repair World Journal of Surgery, 31:421-422, 2007.

Are the Groin Nerves Important to Me?

None of these nerves are functionally important. *They do not control motor function. They do not control erection or ejaculation. They do not give sensation to the penis or clitoris.*

Once this is understood, it remains to identify which nerve is the source of pain and develop a strategy to remove this injured nerve.

Where is the Groin?

Where exactly is your groin and what nerves are involved? Figure 4-1 shows the area from the front of your hip bone (anterior superior iliac crest) to your inner thigh, which includes your pubic area. The different colors are anatomic areas that related to four different nerves. Each of these nerves can be injured by an operation. The operative site is shown as a scar.

It is important to understand that the nerves to the groin begin inside the pelvis, come around the inside of the abdominal wall to enter the skin. These nerves can be injured by surgery that is done along the pathway of the nerve.

The pain is felt in the skin innervated by the nerve. The scar can be painful because that is where the nerve is injured, and this is considered as the trigger spot for the pain. As an example, touching the hernia scar may cause the pain which is perceived to come from the inner thigh skin. The thigh skin itself might be numb, or might be painful when touched.

In the approach that I developed, a new incision is made near the iliac crest, the "hip pointer" area (Fig 4-17). I do not go through the old scar. The small nerves causing the pain can be identified here and relocated out of the abdominal wall, and put back into the pelvic area where they arise.

Hysterectomy and Abdominoplasty

Harriet D. needed to have a hysterectomy.

She had gained sufficient weight that at age 55 she had a larger bulging lower abdomen than she wished. She did not like how she appeared in tight clothes. So her Gynecologist referred her to a Plastic Surgeon. He agreed that her abdominal musculature was weak, and that she had sufficient excess skin that she would appear much improved if he tightened her abdominal wall muscles and removed the excess skin. He explained this would leave an incision longer than the Gynecologist would have left for the hysterectomy alone, and she would also have a scar around her belly button (umbilicus). The "makeover" plan was therefore to do a hysterectomy and an abdomino-plasty at the same operation.

Harriet agreed. The surgery went without a problem. Harriet awoke with a feeling of tightness in her lower abdomen, as expected.

Two weeks later Harriet noticed that her abdomen did not feel tight any longer. But the incision on the right side was opening due to a localized infection, and her right thigh was numb. Her thigh became painful when she would sit. Her scar became thick and painful when touched (see Figure 4-4).

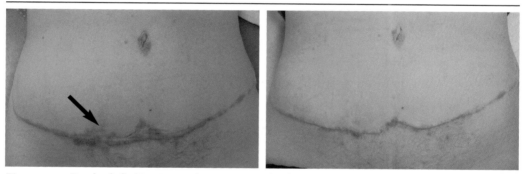

Figure 4-4. On the left, Harriet is shown 4 months following her abdominoplasty and hysterectomy combined procedure. There were wound healing problems on the right side, as noted by the thickened scar. The arrow shows the site at which the scar was painful due to a neuroma of the ilioinguinal nerve. Her condition after a Dellon-designed procedure is shown on the right. This appearance is at 14 days following scar excision, removal of the painful ilioinguinal nerve, and neurolysis of the lateral femoral cutaneous nerve (which causes numbness in the blue region shown in Figure 4-2 above). This surgery immediately relieved her pain and improved her appearance cosmetically at the same time.

Harriet's Plastic Surgeon referred her to me. He was aware of my research into groin pain, and the fact that the small nerves of the abdominal wall can become damaged by scar and cause groin pain.* He also was aware, through my writings in the Plastic Surgery literature,** that entrapment of a nerve near the hip bone can cause numbness in the front and side of the thigh.

I saw Harriet 7 months after her "makeover." From her complaints, of a painful scar, it was clear that she had a neuroma of the ilioinguinal nerve, and possibly also the iliohypogastric nerve, since the first surgical procedure went high up on the abdominal wall. Nothing further was required in terms of testing to determine this then to do the physical examination, which identified the painful area of the scar in the area that had opened (see Figure 4-1). X-rays do not show these small nerves, even the newest MRI can not show these nerves, which are just 1or 2 mm in size.

It was clear from Harriet's complaints that the front of thigh bothered her, and was made worse with sitting. I believed she might also have compression of the lateral femoral cutaneous nerve (LFC), the nerve next to the hip bone (blue color in Figure 4-1). To document this, she had neurosensory testing with the Pressure-Specified Sensory Device™ (PSSD) This is a painless test, using a computer-linked measurement of pressure perception. In fact, I invented the PSSD in 1989 in order to be able to measure the function of the sensory nerves for problems such as this (more on the PSSD in Chapter 1, on Neuroma, Nerve Compression & Neuropathy).

---

*Liszka, TG, Dellon, AL, Manson PN; Iliohypogastric nerve entrapment following abdomino-plasty. Plastic Reconstructive Surgery; 93: 181- 183, 1994.

**Nahabedian, MY, Dellon, AL, Meralgia paresthetica: Etiology, diagnosis, and outcome of surgical decompression, Annals Plastic Surgery, 35:590-594, 1995.

Harriet's test result, shown in Figure 4-5. It demonstrated no two-point discrimination in the right thigh region innervated by this nerve. This meant that the LFC was dying. A neurolysis or the LFC was needed.

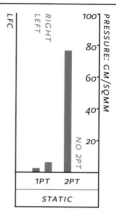

Figure 4-5. Harriet's neurosensory testing result. The Pressure-Specified Sensory Device™ demonstrated no right (red) two-point discrimination (2PT) in the region of the right lateral femoral cutaneous (LFC) nerve. There is still some function of this nerve as demonstrated by the normal height of the red one-point static touch (1PT). This documents a severe degree of nerve compression. The left side (blue) documents normal measurements.

I operated on Harriet, removing the previously poorly healed scar, removing the two nerves to the skin that were responsible for her pain, the ilioinguinal and iliohypogastric nerves, and saving the lateral femoral cutaneous nerve by doing a neurolysis.

Harriet awoke from this operation knowing that her thigh had its usual feeling restored. When she touched her previously painful scar the next day, it no longer hurt. She was better. The appearance of her abdomen is shown in Figure 4-4 (right) at the time of her suture removal, 14 days after the surgery.

Gastric By-Pass and Abdominoplasty

In the year 2005, it was estimated by the American College of Surgeons that there will be 120,000 surgical procedures performed to help people lose weight. Surgery to lose weight is called bariatric surgery.

Gastric by-pass surgery, or gastric stapling are forms of bariatric surgery that reduce the capacity of the stomach to hold food.

Being severely overweight threatens life itself. Bariatric surgery is successful in accomplishing significant weight loss in most patients. Like all surgery, there are potential complications.

Probably the most natural outcome of this surgery is that the skin cannot shrink up, leaving loose, hanging skin, especially in the abdomen. As noted for the patient described above, Harriet, Plastic Surgery can reduce this excessive skin. For Harriet, a traditional abdominoplasty was needed. After gastric by-pass, with loss of 100 pounds or more, skin must be removed from both the horizontal dimension (as Harriet had done) and from the vertical dimension, as Sandra needed to have done (see Figure 4-6).

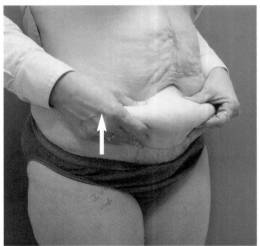 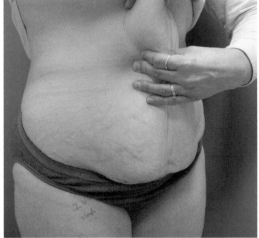

Figure 4-6. Sandra, after loosing 145 pounds, 1.5 years after gastric by-pass surgery. Left: shows vertical excess skin. Right: The horizontal excess skin that can be removed by a Fleur-de-Lys abdominoplasty, described by A. Lee Dellon, MD in 1985.* The arrow points to the site of her groin pain related to insertion of the caval umbrella.

*Dellon AL: Fleur-de-lis abdominoplasty. Aesthetic Plast Surg 9:27-32, 1985.

Another complication of being overweight and having bariatric surgery, is the risk of a blood clot forming in the leg, and then moving into the lung. This deep vein thrombosis and subsequent pulmonary embolism can be life threatening. For this reason, at some centers for bariatric surgery, a thin, metal "umbrella" is inserted into the vena cava, the large vein bringing blood to the heart from the legs. This caval umbrella is inserted through the large femoral blood vessels in the groin.

Sandra's pain began when the umbrella was inserted through her right groin into her vena cava. The pain went into her inner thigh, and stayed there. She was told it would go away. The next day she had her gastric by-pass surgery (see Figure 4-7).

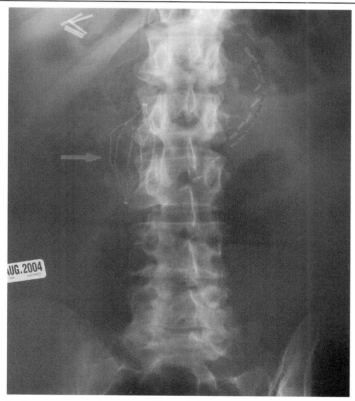

Figure 4-7. Sandra's post-operative x-ray of her abdomen demonstrates the curved row of staples on her stomach (red dashed line), and the "umbrella" placed into her vena cava to prevent blood clots from reaching her heart (red arrow). Vascular clips are upper right. The metal umbrella was placed through her right groin, injuring a nerve.

Sandra's by-pass was successful. In 18 months she lost almost half her weight, going from 290 pounds to 135 pounds. But she remained in pain.

Sandra required narcotic medication for her right groin pain. She was prevented from enjoying the new thinner self she had become because of her constant pain. She was unable to play with her children or enjoy activities with her husband.

I operated on Sandra to relieve her of the groin pain by removing the damaged nerve. At the same time, I did her abdominoplasty.

Sandra awoke without the groin pain that had prevented her carrying out even the regular activities of her daily life. And she loved the appearance of her new abdomen too (Figure 4-8).

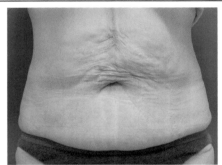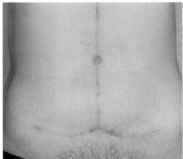

Figure 4-8: Sandra. Left: before surgery. Right: 6 weeks after a Fleur-de-lis abdominoplasty that improved the appearance of her abdomen after gastric by-pass surgery. Surgical exposure used to remove excess skin also allowed removal of the damaged nerve that caused her groin pain.

Painful Scar after Hysterectomy

Gynecologists are experts at operating on pelvic problems for women.

Gynecologists make the low, "bikini cut" incision hundreds of thousands of times a year in the United States. It is done for hysterectomy. It is done for Caesarian sections (to deliver babies). It is used for bladder suspensions for urinary incontinence. This incision is well-hidden and usually painless. Many Gynecologists have not had a painful scar.

The ilioinguinal nerve and the iliohypogastric nerve can send branches into this area to innervate the lower abdominal wall and the pubic, hair bearing, skin.

I have helped relieve pain in many women who have pain in these scars. Usually, I must remove both of these nerves. Examples are given in Figure 4-9 and 4-10 below.

The surgery is performed with a general anesthetic. The surgery takes about one hour for each side. The pain is gone usually upon awakening. Normal activities can be resumed the second day. The sutures are removed on the 12th to 14th day. The inner thigh, pubic hair area, and lower abdominal wall will have abnormal sensation, but it may not be much different than what you have.

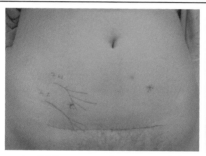
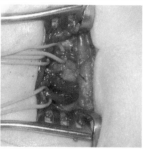

Figure 4-9. The typical Pfannenstiel incision (bikini cut) is shown above. It is the type used for hysterectomy and for Cesarian-section. This incision can be a source of pain. Left: The pathways for the ilioinguinal (I.I.) and for the iliohypogastric (I.H.) nerves is shown going towards the scar. An old, pale, appendectomy scar is noted. The asterisks are trigger spots for the I.H. nerve, which is injured bilaterally (both sides) in this patient. Right: The incision is opened and the blue plastic loops show the I.H. (top) and the I.I. (bottom) nerves going into the scar.

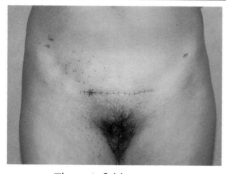
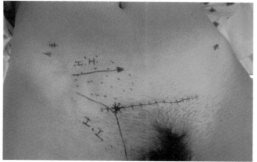

Figure 4-10. The painful hysterectomy scar. Left: The areas of numbness in the inner thigh, typically supplied by the ilioinguinal nerve, and that in the lower abdominal wall typically supplied by the iliohypogastric nerve. The asterisk in the incision is the trigger spot. The other small scars are sites where an endoscope punctured the skin to treat endometriosis. Right: The arrows show the pathways of the I.H. and I.I. nerves.

Testicular Pain after Orchiectomy

Removal of the testicle is called an orchiectomy. The thought alone is painful. The testicle may be removed for cancer or chronic infection.

When the testicle is removed, its nerve, the genital branch of the genitofemoral nerve (GF) must be cut. If a person perceives pain in the testicle, that pain is transmitted by this nerve.

The GF nerves exits the abdominal wall with the spermatic cord.

The GF nerve can be injured doing a hernia repair, because it is in the external inguinal ring, along with the ilioinguinal nerve and the hernia sac.

When the GF nerve is injured, the person complains of pain in the testicle. He does not complain of pain in the thigh or groin unless the ilioinguinal nerve is also injured. Which it often is.

Women do not have testicles. Women have ovaries.

Women do have a GF nerve. It goes to the inside of the labia majora, the vulva. It does not go to the vagina.

The underside of the scrotum is not innervated by the GF nerve, but rather by the perineal branches of the pudendal nerve. This nerve also innervates the external part of the vagina. The pudendal nerve exists between the legs, near the rectum, and is not in the groin.

James had just had 11 operations in 16 months.

At the first operation, his left testicle was removed. He had been treated by the best Urologists and Infectious disease specialists. His chronic infections of the small tubes around the testicle (epididymitis) could not be stopped. His profession as a motivational speaker had been on hold. His wife and three children were as supportive as possible.

James had severe, constant pain in his left testicle, even though he did not have a left testicle anymore.

One of his specialists thought a hernia was present. He had the hernia repaired with mesh. His pain spread to include his inner thigh.

He had the mesh removed.

He had a bleeding problem into the hernia site after removing the mesh. The blood had to be drained. Then this area became infected, and his wound had to be drained again.

James went to a Pain Management doctor. Local anesthetic was injected into his spine (epidural catheter) on several occasions. This was done in the operating room each time. He was even admitted to the hospital and the catheter was left in place for several days in his spine.

James became addicted to narcotics and unable to work.

Finally, the Pain Management specialist suggest that James have a spinal cord stimulator placed. This mean putting an electrical stimulator into James' spine, running the electrical cord around to the front of his belly, and implanting a small metal and plastic computer into his body. This helped a little. He went back to surgery to have the stimulator "repositioned" in his spine (see Chapter 10 on Stimulators). It did not really help him very much. He continued his medications.

And finally, the stimulator in the front of his belly became infected. Its pouch was drained. Then they had to remove the stimulator so that the infection did not spread along the wire into the spine. He was left with an open wound on his abdomen, which was to close slowly on its own over several months.

Have you lost count yet?

Mary, James' wife, found me on the internet. "Can you help us?" she asked. "We live in Virginia. I believe my husband can make the trip."

"I can help you," I replied. "Come on up!"

At the time I saw James, Figure 4-11 (left) is the appearance of his groin and abdomen. The drain is in the open wound which previously had held his spinal stimulator. He could point directly to the spot near his pubic bone where pain radiated to the testicle. He came prepared for surgery the next day, in case I could really help him. I had held a 2 hour space for James on my operating schedule in case I could help him.

"I can fix this for you James," I said. At surgery, the genital branch of the genitofemoral nerve was at the external ring, where the Urologist had removed the testicle, and where the mesh and infection had been (Fig 4-12).

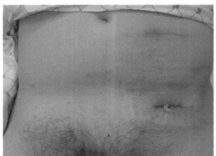
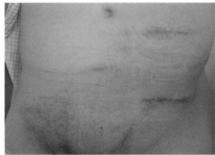

Figure 4-11. After 11 operations in 16 months, James, who first had his left testicle removed, has testicular pain localized at the red dot (Left) and a rubber drain in his abdominal wound where his spinal cord stimulator had been located. On the Right, 4 weeks after removal of the genitofemoral nerve through the pubic incision, removal of the ilioinguinal and iliohy-pogastric nerves through the incision near the hip bone, which was also used to excise the non-healing wound, the spinal cord stimulator site.

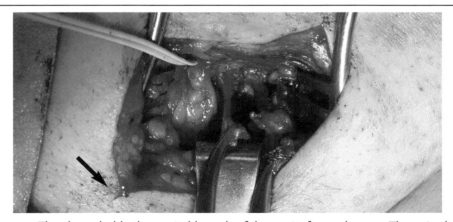

Figure 4-12. The clamp holds the genital branch of the genitofemoral nerve. The pain that signals testicular pain. The black arrow can be matched to red dot in Figure 4-11 at left.

James awoke from surgery without testicular pain.

James and Mary spent that night in the hotel across from the hospital, and I saw them the next morning. He had no bleeding. His wound was remaining closed. He had no more testicular pain. His scars no longer hurt.

James and Mary returned to see me 4 weeks later. He had no more testicular pain. His scar did not hurt. His wound remained closed (Figure 4-11 right). He had already switched from narcotics to anti-inflammatories, and was reducing his Neurontin dose. James is 60 years old. He had returned to work. Mary was happy too.

On November 16, 2005, I had this e-mail from James:

"Doctor Dellon, thank you. I am off all drugs and have resumed my regular activities and motivational speaking. Yesterday I walked 6 miles, and I ached a little. It is just 4 months since surgery. Am I doing too much? Before your operation I had terrible pain with intercourse and had lost most of my sexual function and desire. *Full function has returned, and it is like I am in my twenties again. Once again, sex is all fun and no pain (and several times per week). You have helped me beyond measure.* Please tell people my story. It should give hope to others."

Cardiac Catheterization Caused Groin Pain

The exact number of cardiac catheterizations done each year in the United States must exceed half a million. It is likely that one of these will injure a nerve during placement of the catheter into the groin. Here is just one person to whom this happened.

Janis (not her real name) is a nurse in Ohio. She had chest pain one day at work. She had an EKG which was normal. Her cardiologist was worried, as Janis was under a lot of stress in her work and personal life. A near, dear relative had recently died. Janis was 52 years old. The Cardiologist sent Janis for a "stress EKG" test. As she was running on the treadmill, Janis had chest pain, although the EKG did not change. Faced with this puzzle, the Cardiologist felt it was best for Janis to have a cardiac catheterization.

During this test, done in the hospital, in a special Radiology Cardiac Center, using sterile technique, like a real operation, the Cardiologist or Radiologist insert a large metal needle into the femoral artery in the right groin. Through this, a small catheter is inserted all the way to the heart. Then x-ray dye is put in and a picture of the arteries of the heart is obtained.

Janis has a normal heart.

Janis now had groin pain.

The following pathway is now well known to you. Janis could point to a spot in her groin that set off the pain. The Cardiologist and Radiologist never had seen this problem before. Topical pain medication to the spot relieved the pain. Janis could not take narcotics and still function as a nurse. Janis had side effects from the non-narcotic, neuropathic pain medications, like Neurontin. Two years after her cardiac catheterization, Janis was sent by Pain Management to have a spinal cord stimulator placed.

The location of Janis's pain is shown in Figure 4-13. A picture of her back with its five incisions for placement of her stimulators is shown in Chapter 10 on Stimulators (Figure 10-3).

I operated on Janis, removing the femoral branch of the genitofemoral nerve. It was the source of her pain. She is pain free.

Her spinal cord stimulator has been removed.

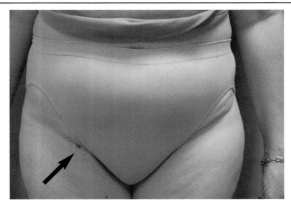

Figure 4-13. Arrow and blue dot mark the site of pain remaining 3 years after a cardiac catheterization. A spinal cord stimulator was placed, moved, and replaced. What was needed was removal of the painful neuroma.

Ileostomy and Groin Pain

When the intestine must be brought out on to the abdominal wall, the possibility of pain related to one of the nerves to the groin is real. It is unusual, but it is real. I have two patients with this problem. *How many more people are out there with groin pain after ileostomy or colostomy?*

Marcia (not her real name) is 75 years old. She is mentally sharp as a tack. She dresses beautifully. Her hair always looks like she has just come from the beauty parlor. A husband Marty (not his real name) is a lively 78. He will only have health care administered by the best people. Which in his view, is always someone trained at Johns Hopkins. He is a benefactor.

Her bladder cancer was treated with radiation therapy at a time when the exact dose to kill the cancer was not really known. That was 28 years ago. Her Hopkins Gynecologic Oncologist removed her bladder and uterus. The radiation killed the remaining cancer cells. It also killed part of her intestine. And so she had an ileostomy.

She is happy she is alive.

Then the radiation killed the skin of her lower abdomen. Plastic Surgeons at Johns Hopkins removed the dead skin, muscle and connective tissue. They then created a new lower abdomen for Marcia from the skin and muscle of her right leg. Plastic mesh was also required to strengthen the large abdominal wall defect. When the flap was moved from the leg to the abdomen, it required a point of rotation in her right groin, The flap lived (see Figure 4-14). The abdominal wall and thigh were both closed again.

Marcia's groin pain started shortly thereafter. The pain went from just below her ileostomy to the right groin, and into her thigh. She went to Pain Management doctors in Pennsylvania, trying to get relief.
Her pain persisted for one year.

Finally she received my name from her Gynecologic Oncologist, the one who had saved her life with her initial tumor. He was from Johns Hopkins Hospital. He knew me. Indeed, he and I were residents together at Johns Hopkins Hospital in the late 1970's. He knew of my interest in nerves.

Marcia saw me. Marty was with her. She could hardly climb on to the examining table because of pain. She could hardly lie down flat to be examined. She felt much better if her leg was bent at the hip. I found her to have a trigger spot, below the ileostomy, near the iliohypogastric nerve. There was a trigger spot for the ilioinguinal nerve as well. Her entire front and side of her thigh had burning pain when the skin was touched.

"I can help you, Marcia," I said. We need to remove three nerves. They have been stretched and caught in scar tissue by the flap.

"I will gladly trade numbness for pain," Marcia said.

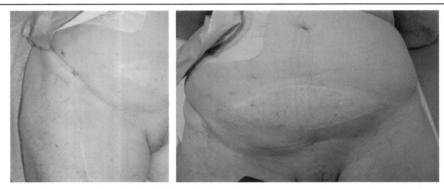

Figure 4-14. Marcia's right thigh (left), with long healed scar at the site where the leg muscle and skin were taken as a flap and rotated to reconstruct the lower abdominal wall (right). On the left, note the area of thigh pain outlined in blue, indicating damage to the lateral femoral cutaneous nerve. Near the ileostomy bag, not the trigger spots where the iliohypogastric and ilioinguinal nerves were caught in the flap rotation.

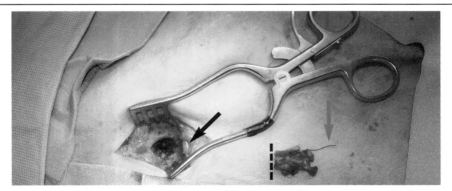

Figure 4-15. Marcia, intra-operative view. Note blue suture (blue arrow) attached to piece of mesh (dashed line) and the damaged lateral femoral cutaneous nerve (LFC, black arrow). The dark opening is the space the LFC nerve came through, and into which it was placed back inside the abdominal cavity.

At surgery, the lateral femoral cutaneous nerve was stuck in scar tissue to the mesh by a suture (Figure 4-15). The nerve was divided and dropped into her abdomen. The iliohypogastric and ilioinguinal nerves were also removed.

Two months after the surgery, Marcia and Marty came back to see me from Pennsylvania. Marcia said, "My pain is gone. My life is worth living again."

Marty said, "My brother has knee pain after his knee replacement. Can you help him?"

"Yes," I said (see Chapter 3 on Knee Pain).

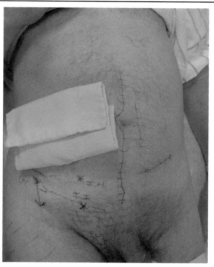

Figure 4-16. Another example of groin pain associated with ileostomy. A 48 year old man four years after bowel resection for ulcerative colitis. Has had many previous abdominal operations for his bowel problems. The bag can be seen on his ileostomy. He has numbness in the thigh, but not pain, and his lateral femoral cutaneous nerve can be saved with a neurolysis. His iliohypogastric nerve (I.H. trigger point) and ilioinguinal nerve (I.I. trigger point) will require resection of these nerves. He has come to the Dellon Institutes for Peripheral Nerve Surgery® from Holland, upon referral from the Chief of Plastic Surgery, Moshe Kon, in Utrecht. Dr Kon knew of my interest in peripheral nerves.

How many Nerves should be Removed?

From the above examples, I have tried to convey the complexity of deciding what to do for the patient with groin pain. The answer is not as simple as "always do a triple nerve resection."

When the patient comes to me for a consultation, I listen to their exact complaints and learn where, during my physical examination, the trigger points for their pain are located.

There are four nerves to be considered. Usually the lateral femoral cutaneous nerve can be saved, but sometimes, as with Marcia (above), it may be so damaged that it must be removed. The genital branch of the genitofemoral nerve does not have to be removed unless there is clearly testicular pain present. Almost always, the ilioinguinal and iliohypogastric nerves must be removed. Figure 4-17 show two examples of patients who each only needed the ilioinguinal and iliohypogastric nerves removed.

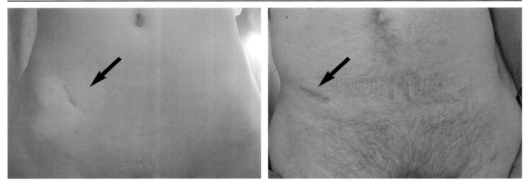

Figure 4-17. Examples of typical incision near the anterior superior iliac crest (black arrows) used to remove the ilioinguinal and iliohypogastric nerves.

Complex Groin Pain Patients

In the patient in Figure 4-18, the number of incisions in the abdomen speaks for itself. I was able to relieve this patient of pain by excision of the ilioinguinal and iliohypogastric nerves. This patient's iliohypogastric nerve can be seen clearly.

Groin pain patients are complex, and each must be considered as an individual, and an individual surgical plan arrived at together.

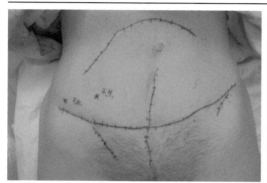
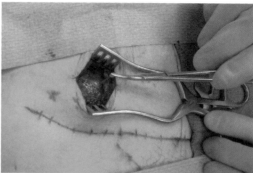

Figure 4-18. Right groin pain in 60 year old woman who has had many surgeries. Pain was relieved by resecting the ilioinguinal and iliohypogastric (held in clamp) nerves.

As a final example, consider the patient shown in Figure 4-19. He is a 26 year old man who has had bilateral inguinal hernia repairs. Mesh was used bilaterally. He has bilateral groin pain, worse on the left than on the right. He can point to his areas of pain, which are noted in the photographs. He did have left testicular pain. His surgery required ilioinguinal and iliohypogastric nerves to be removed bilaterally, He also needed the left genital branch of the genitofemoral nerve removed.

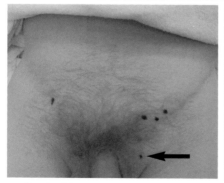
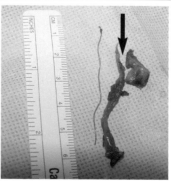

Figure 4-19. Left: The black dots indicate trigger points for the pain. On the left side, note the black dot over the spermatic cord in the pubic hair (arrow). This was the trigger spot for the genital branch of the genitofemoral nerve. Right: The nerve has been removed. It was found to have the blue suture connecting it to the mesh. Note the notch (arrow) in the mesh, which caused the testicular pain.

Tack this on at the End

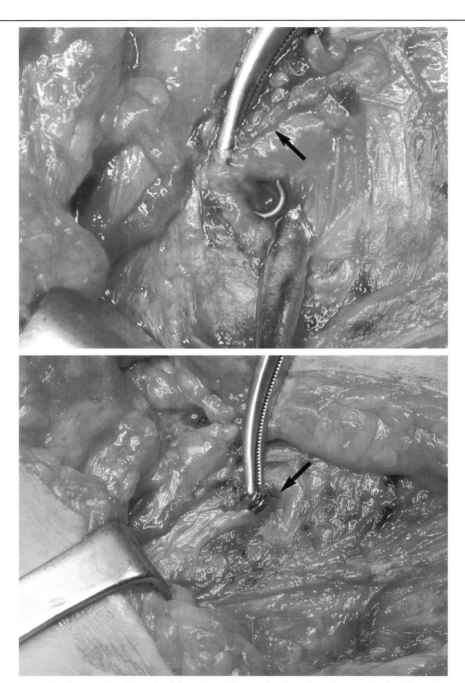

Figure 4-20. Mesh repair of inguinal hernia with mesh placed endoscopically. Top: The metal tack is noted encircling the ilioinguinal nerve and mesh (arrow). Bottom: The metal tack is held in clamp. The nerve is held in the tack (arrow).

Pain Solutions Summary

Groin pain after surgery or injury can be due to a nerve.

There are four different nerves that may contribute to your pain.

If it is more than 6 months from the time of your last surgery, and if medication and other therapy measures have not relieved your pain, then the solution to your groin pain problem most likely involves removing one or more of the nerves that are causing your pain.

Where can I learn more about Groin Pain?

On the internet, the Dellon Institute for Peripheral Nerve Surgery® website has more information and a BROCHURE on *Groin Pain* that can be downloaded at http://www.dellon.com

You can call the HOTLINE at +1 877-DELLON-1 (+1 877-335-5661).

5

Chapter Five
Thoracic Outlet Syndrome

"I cannot control my shoulder. I cannot hold my right arm over my head. My fingers now go numb, and my shoulder aches."

Winging It

Bruce (not his real name) is a strong man, with serious, piercing eyes. He is tall and handsome. Bruce has been working as a lineman for the telephone company for ten years. He likes to climb telephone poles and fix the overhead wires. Today, as he speaks to me, he is intense, and frustrated.

"Doctor Dellon", Bruce explains, "that is exactly my problem. I cannot control my shoulder. I cannot hold my right arm over my head. My fingers now go numb, and my shoulder aches. The last doctor looked at my back and told me that my shoulder blade was sticking out. He said I have a 'winged scapula' and that I am becoming paralyzed! Can you help me?"

"Yes Bruce, I can help you," I said. "Tell me how this began. Did you injure yourself somehow?"

"Yes, Doctor Dellon, I did. I was pulling broken tree branches away from a telephone pole after a storm, trying to restore power. I was dragging the tree limb behind me, when I felt a sudden tearing pain in the right side of my neck and pain went into my shoulder. I dropped the large tree branch, and the pain slowly went away. But I could not use my arm properly. I went right in to the company doctor that day. He took x-rays and examined my arm, but found nothing wrong. The next day I went back to work. I could work, but the aching in my shoulder and problems with the use of my right arm have never gone away. And they have gotten worse."

"How long ago was that injury," I asked.

"More than two years ago. For the past year I can only work in doors. I cannot do my regular job. I have had lots of therapy. The Orthopedic Surgeon says my rotator cuff is fine and so are the discs in my neck. They did all those special MRI x-rays. When the last doctor found my shoulder blade sticking out, he sent me for one of those EMG tests, where they stick you with needles. You have the report. It shows my muscle is dying, the one that controls my shoulder blade. Can you help me?"

"Yes Bruce," I reassured him, "this is a very unusual problem, but I can fix it for you. It is called, as you have said, a winged scapula. The shoulder blade sticks out because the nerve to the muscle that controls the shoulder blade had been injured. That nerve is part of the brachial plexus, a collection of nerves that controls all upper extremity movement, including the shoulder. You have brachial plexus compression, but before I discus this with you further, Let me show you a picture in the anatomy book to explain this complex area better to you." (See Figures 5-1 and 5-2.)

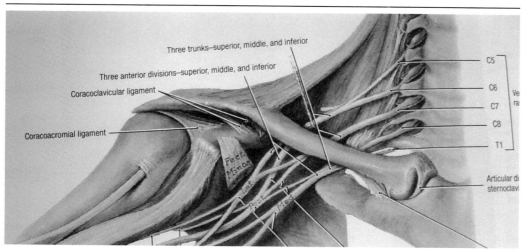

Figure 5-1. Traditional anatomy drawing of the right brachial plexus. The five cervical nerve roots (C5,C6,C7,C8, and T1, shown in yellow) are depicted without a muscle covering and the long thoracic nerve, responsible for winging of the scapula is not shown.

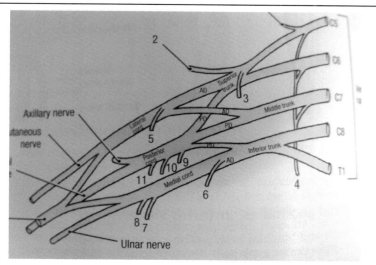

Figure 5-2. Traditional schematic of the brachial plexus which shows the nerves intertwining without showing the muscles or bones. This schematic shows the long thoracic nerve as nerve number 4, going downwards and into the region of the chest cavity, which is NOT where this nerve actually goes.

I explained that in many forms of injury, the small muscles that help in turning the head and protruding the chin, such as when you are working at the computer or after a "whiplash" injury from a car accident, become trapped by the scarring or spasm of these muscles. As can be seen in Figures 5-1 and 5-2, this small region contains all the nerves to the neck, shoulder, part of the chest, and the entire arm. Therefore the symptoms that a patient can have range from just the winging of the scapula to numbness and weakness of the entire arm, chest or breast pain, neck pain, and headaches that are in the back of the head on the same side as the shoulder pain. The symptoms are all made worse when the arm is held in the air, over the head.

This entire collection of symptoms can be so vague as to make the doctor think that there cannot be a single cause for it. Unfortunately, the degree of compression is often mild enough that the traditional evaluation

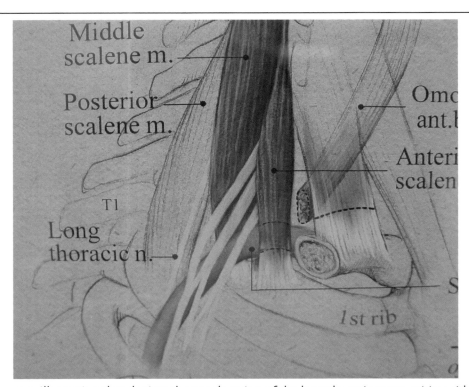

Figure 5-3. Illustration that depicts the true location of the long thoracic nerve exiting either beneath or between the scalene muscles. In this location, the nerve can become stuck by a torn, injured muscle. In this location the nerve can be identified and reconstructed. (With permission http://www.dellon.com)

by the neurologist and orthopedic surgeon do not find anything wrong. Because this symptom complex occurs frequently in the setting of a car accident or workmen's compensation, the patient often is not believed, and thought to be malingering.

About 50 years ago, this symptom complex was called "Scalenus Anticus Syndrome," and when doctors thought of this diagnosis, they understood that this muscle, the anterior scalene, needed to be removed.

In Figure 5-3, you can see the long thoracic nerve, and you can see how spasm and scarring of the anterior scalene muscle can compress this group of large important nerves to create all of these symptoms. In 1956, a Physical Therapist from the Mayo Clinic devised exercises to stretch this tight muscle, and strengthen other shoulder muscles like the trapezius and rhomboids, so pressure is lifted from the compressed nerves. In 1956 the name Thoracic Outlet Syndrome was created for this syndrome. While this is a "nice name" it is anatomically incorrect (the thoracic outlet is the diaphragm and this region is properly called the thoracic inlet) and this name thoracic outlet syndrome diverted doctors' attention away from the scalene muscles.

The good news is that 90% of patients will have their symptoms improve with 6 months of therapy described above. If the symptoms do not go away, then surgery can be done to remove the pressure from the brachial plexus.

I believe the correct name for this symptom complex should be "Compression of the Brachial Plexus in the Thoracic Inlet," and while that is a lot of words for a name, it describes the pathology so that a proper operation can be designed to decompress the nerves. I created this name in 1993.* Many doctors believe you should remove the first rib through the armpit (axilla) to correct this problem, but in my experience, the rib does not need to be removed. My approach is located just above the collar bone.

---

*Dellon AL: "Brachial plexus compression" (not "thoracic outlet syndrome"): Treatment by supraclavicular plexus neurolysis. J Reconstr Microsurg 9:11-18, 1993.

Removing the first rib through the armpit has many complications associated with it such as collapse of the lung, injury to the major artery and vein to the arm, and injury to the nerves to the skin of the armpit, creating more pain whenever the arm is elevated. Figure 5-4 shows an example of this complication. Furthermore, often a small piece of rib is left that still causes compression, and the scalene muscle is still stuck to the nerves.

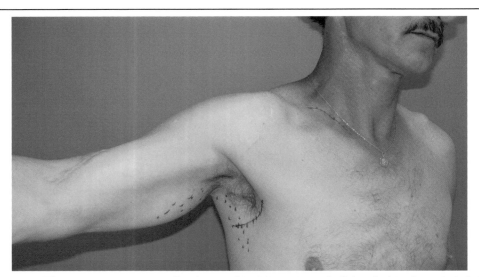

Figure 5-4. This man is two years after having his "thoracic outlet" (really his thoracic inlet) decompressed by removing his first rib through his armpit. This surgery failed to help him, and left him with the area under his arm and on his chest that is painful to touch (shown in blue dots); a neuroma of the second intercosto-brachial nerve. I can still help him by removing this damaged nerve, and then operating along the blue line near his collar bone to remove his anterior scalene muscle and decompress his brachial plexus.

The surgical approach that I favor requires an incision in the neck near the collar bone. The surgery is done under general anesthesia. Because my surgery is done with microsurgical technique, and because the rib is left in place, I have excellent control over the nerves, blood vessels, and lungs. This surgery is successful in 80% of patients, relieving pain and permitting them to use the hand and arm in the overhead position again, as is demonstrated in Figure 5-5.

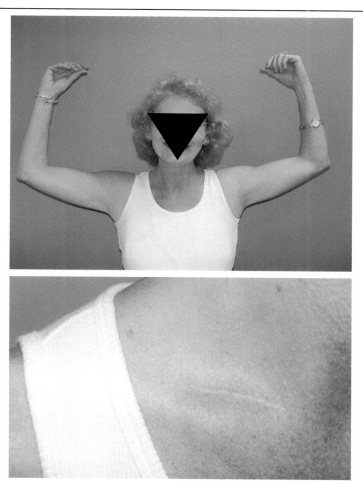

Figure 5-5. Top: Woman who is one year after my supraclavicular brachial plexus neurolysis. She is smiling as her symptoms are relieved, and demonstrates holding her hands overhead. Bottom: Note appearance of the scar at one year.

"Thank you Dr. Dellon for explaining that to me." It is very complicated. But do you have any pictures you can show to me of someone with my degree of muscle paralysis who is better?"

"Bruce," I replied, "yes, I do. And there is hope for you too." (See Figure 5-6.)

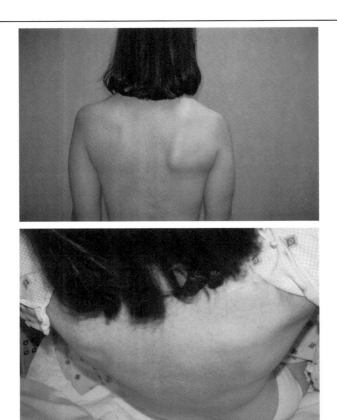

Figure 5-6. A young woman injured left shoulder while being twirled by her dancing partner 6 months ago. The winging of the right scapula is present (top) even without trying to lift her right arm. She can elevate her right arm (bottom) in the recovery room following the surgical procedure.

I described the entrapment for the long thoracic nerve in the year 1999, and reported my first five cases of successful surgery with two of our Johns Hopkins Plastic Surgery residents in 2001.*

"I am ready for the surgery Doctor Dellon," said Bruce. "Are there any more tests you need to do for me?" (See Figure 5-7.)

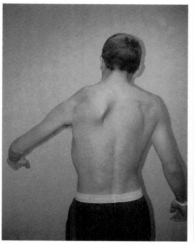 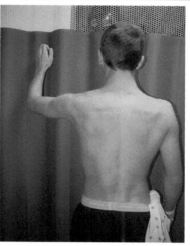

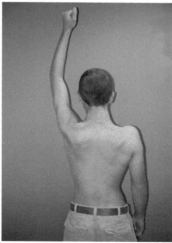

Figure 5-7. Top Left: The young man, injured wrestling 6 months before, was unable to lift his right arm higher than shown. The "chicken bone" or winged scapula is clearly seen protruding from his back. Top Right: He is shown still in the hospital the day after surgery. He can now lift his arm higher and already the serratus anterior muscle is pulling the scapula back against the rib cage, correcting the winging. Bottom: Three weeks after surgery.

*Disa J, Wang B, Dellon AL: Correction of scapular winging by neurolysis of the long thoracic nerve. J Reconstructive Microsurgery, 17: 79-84, 2001.

"Bruce, not for you. Most people with symptoms of 'thoracic outlet syndrome' do not have winging. They have a lot of complaints in their hands. For those people I do a neurosensory test with the Pressure-Specified Sensory Device™, which documents abnormal sensory nerve function when the hand is at rest, and then after the hand has been held elevated for 3 minutes. This type of testing puts additional compression on the brachial plexus, and helps us determine whether the patient will benefit from more therapy, whether they need a neurolysis of their brachial plexus (an anterior scalenectomy), or whether they have some other problem with their arm like compression of the ulnar nerve at the elbow, called 'cubital tunnel syndrome.' This is compression of the ulnar nerve at the site where you strike your 'funny bone and feel it shoot into your little finger." (See Figure 5-8.)

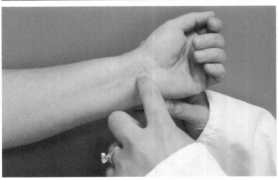 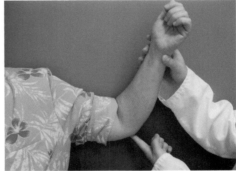

Figure 5-8. Entrapment of peripheral nerves, like the median nerve at the wrist(left), causing carpal tunnel syndrome, or ulnar nerve entrapment at the elbow (right), causing cubital tunnel syndrome, demonstrated here, can refer symptoms to the neck and shoulder and give symptoms similar to those of brachial plexus compression. If these peripheral nerve are compressed, they should be treated surgically first, as the more proximal neck and shoulder symptoms may also go away. Compression of the ulnar nerve at the elbow can give symptoms of coldness in the hand, but so can compression of the main artery to the arm (see Figure 5-3). If vascular compression is present, it should be decompressed before decompressing the peripheral nerves (see Figure 5-9).

More typical are the complaints of Leslie (not her real name), a 40 year old waitress. "Doctor Dellon", said Leslie, "I can no longer carry trays with my right hand. Not only do all my fingers go numb, but the side of jaw hurts and I have horrible headaches. My dentist told me I have 'TMJ' but my teeth are lined up well. This is getting worse and worse. I now even have trouble just trying to dry my hair. Can you help me?"

"Yes Leslie, I can help you," I said. "In many people, an injury has not occurred. Instead, you most likely were born with either extra muscles that press upon your nerves, or the complicated pattern of the brachial plexus (see Figure 5-1 and 5-2) did not form normally. The muscles pull on the back of your head, where they arise from the first few cervical vertebra, and this causes those headaches. Nerves to the skin at the side of your face come through these muscles too, get compressed, and give facial pain, that is often said to be due to the temporomandibular joint (TMJ). The operation that I do, removal of the extra muscles and the anterior scalene muscle, and removal of scar tissue from the nerves, neurolysis of the brachial plexus, can relieve your symptoms," I said.*

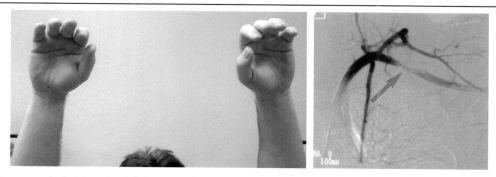

Figure 5-9. Left: Note the left hand is white when elevated compared to the right hand which is more pink. Right: Note the black dye coming from the heart is blocked (arrow) as it tries to flow into the subclavian artery to the right arm while the arm is elevated. This documents vascular compression which can be present in addition to compression of the nerves of the brachial plexus.

*Howard M, Lee C, Dellon AL: Documentation of Brachial Plexus Compression in the thoracic inlet utilizing provocation with Neurosensory and Motor Testing. J Reconstr Microsurg, 19:303-312, 2003.

"You need to have painless neurosensory testing to document the brachial plexus compression" (see Figure 5-10A).

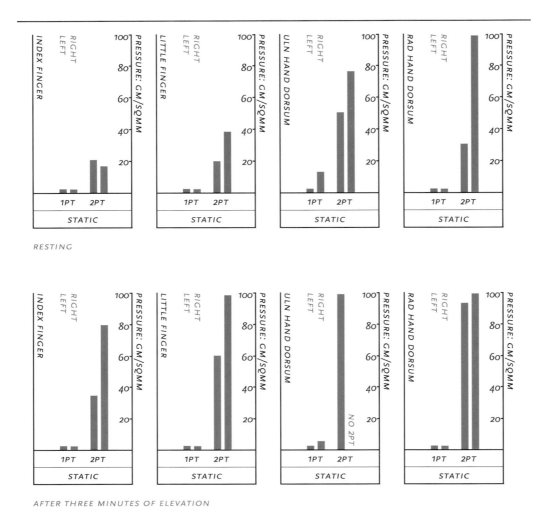

RESTING

AFTER THREE MINUTES OF ELEVATION

Figure 5-10A. Neurosensory with the Pressure-Specified Sensory Device™ done on Leslie prior to surgery. The red bars are the right hand and the blue bars are the left hand. **Higher numbers mean the nerve is not normal.** In the top row, the measurements are taken when the hand is at rest. On the bottom row, the measurements are repeated after the hand has been held up in the air for 3 minutes. Note that on the bottom row, all red bars have gotten higher, and one red bar has disappeared. This documents severe compression of the right brachial plexus, and supports the recommendation for brachial plexus decompression. Note that even the blue bars in the bottom row have become elevated, demonstrating that this waitress is now beginning to have this problem in her left hand too.

Leslie's post-operative neurosensory testing results are shown below (see Figure 5-10B).

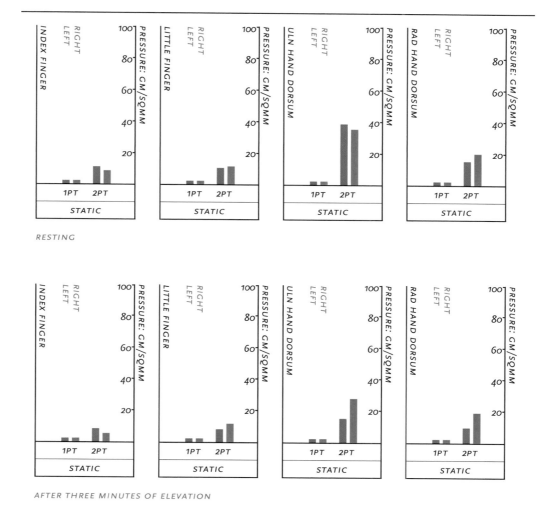

RESTING

AFTER THREE MINUTES OF ELEVATION

Figure 5-10B. The neurosensory testing results after decompressing Leslie's right brachial plexus and removing her anterior scalene muscle, and allowing her left side to rest during the three weeks she was off work. Note that even at rest, both the blue and red bars are lower than they were before surgery. Note that on the bottom row, that now, even with her hand elevated, the blue and red bars no longer increase in height. This documents that pressure has been relieved from the brachial plexus. Her symptoms also were relieved.

After operating on Leslie, I drew a picture of what I found for her parents, who accompanied her to surgery (see Figure 5-11).

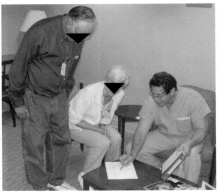

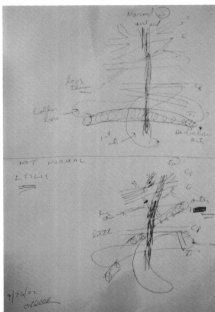

Figure 5-11. Top: After Leslie's operation, Doctor Dellon went out to talk to her parents. Here he is explaining the intra-operative findings to the Leslie's parents. Bottom: Below, is a close-up view of the drawing which shows the normal and the Leslie's anatomical findings. The dark blue is the anterior scalene muscle which was removed. The compressed long thoracic nerve is saved and is shown. The tubular structure is the subclavian artery, which in Leslie was located above the clavicle. The curved structure is the first rib below the clavicle. *The first rib was NOT removed.*

An example of the actual surgery is shown in Figure 5-12.

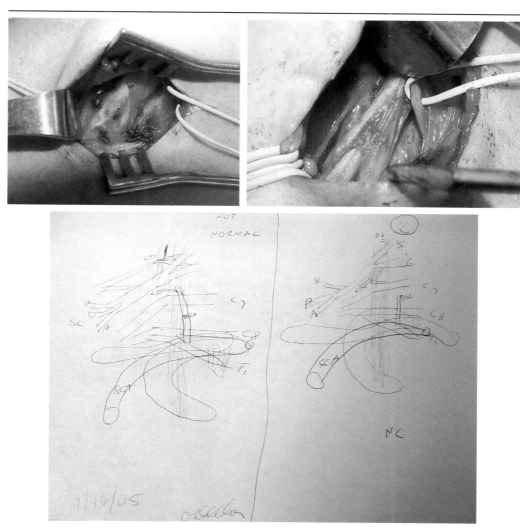

Figure 5-12. Intra-operative photographs of the brachial plexus, with (top left) demonstrating the right scarred upper trunk and suprascapular nerve, which is the source of the shoulder pain and some of the shoulder weakness, and numbness in the thumb and index fingers. The neurolysis of these nerves (top right) has been completed, and the long thoracic nerve has been identified just above and behind this upper trunk. This is the nerve responsible for the scapular winging. The abnormal findings in this patient (bottom), on the left side of the drawing, are contrasted to the normal anatomy on the right. The circular subclavian artery is located in the normal relationship to the clavicle and the curved first rib. The long thoracic nerve (LTN) is drawn in at the top, and may be seen in this location (center) above.

There are those patients who are born with an extra "first rib," which is called a cervical rib, demonstrated in Figure 5-13.

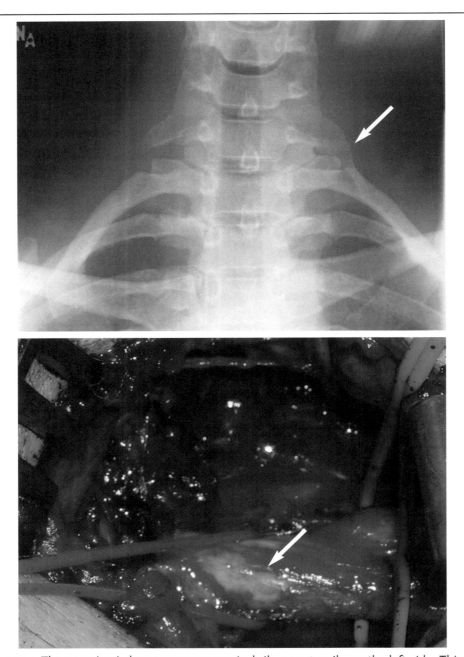

Figure 5-13. The x-ray (top) demonstrates a cervical rib, an extra rib, on the left side. This can cause compression of the brachial plexus and give thoracic outlet symptoms. In this case, that extra rib must be removed. This is shown in surgery (bottom).

Pain Solutions Summary

Five nerves that exit the spine in the neck region combine to form the brachial plexus, the source of all sensory and motor function for the shoulder and hand. If the muscles or other structures in this small region, called the thoracic inlet, become injured, or compressed, the function of the shoulder and hand and the blood vessels that supply them will be changed. This can cause face, neck, shoulder, chest and hand numbness, weakness, and pain, and coldness or swelling in the hand. If the shoulder muscles that hold the scapula to the ribs become weak, this bone sticks out in the back; this is called "winging". Headaches are common.

Most people with these symptoms can be helped by therapy that stretches the tight neck muscle, called the anterior scalene, and strengthens the trapezius and rhomboids that support the shoulder and take pressure away from the brachial plexus. If symptoms persist after 6 months of dedicated therapy, then surgical decompression of the brachial plexus is indicated. My approach for this surgery is through the area just above the collar bone. I remove the tight anterior scalene muscle. I leave the first rib. The relief of upper extremity symptoms and headaches can be dramatic.

Visit Dellon.com or call +1 877-DELLON-1 (+1 877-335-5661) for more information.

6

Chapter Six
Morton's Neuroma
is Not a Neuroma

"Pain shoots into my toe when I step down on the ball of my foot, and I can't wear heels."

Morton's Neuroma

Morton's Neuroma is not a neuroma; it is a nerve entrapment.

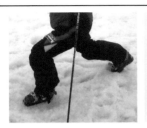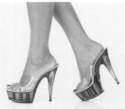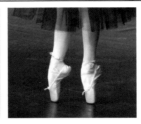

Figure 6-1. Wearing narrow tipped shoes is the leading cause of the chronic entrapment of the interdigital nerve that is known, unfortunately, as Morton's neuroma. Wearing heels makes the problem worse. "Neuroma" is an unfortunate choice of a name for this pain problem. A "neuroma" is "cut out." The problem Morton described in 1876 is now understood to be a nerve entrapment. For a nerve entrapment, the nerve is not cut out.

Philadelphia, 1870's

Thomas G. Morton, MD was an Orthopedic Surgeon at the Philadelphia Orthopedic Hospital and the Pennsylvania Hospital. From 1870 to 1875, Doctor Morton either saw or collected the story of 15 people with what he was to call "A Peculiar and Painful Affection of the Fourth Metatarso-Phalangeal Articulation." Of the 15 people, 13 were women. A few gave a history of an injury to their foot, but most could only say the cause was wearing tight shoes, and three patients had no cause to give at all for their painful fourth toe. He published his observations on this group of patients in 1876.*

Morton never used the term "neuroma" for the cause of his patient's problems. In fact, Morton believed the cause of the pain to be from the *joint* where the 4TH toe joined the foot, the metatarso-phalangeal joint.

Being an Orthopedic Surgeon, and believing the pain came from a joint, Morton operated on 3 of these patients. In two of them, he removed the joint. In the third patient, a Doctor Alison, from Hagerstown, Maryland, Morton amputated the doctor's fourth toe!

Today, about 50,000 nerves are still cut out each year! WHY?

---

*Morton, T.G., A peculiar and painful affection of the fourth metatarso-phalangeal articulation, American Journal of Medical Science, 71:37-45, 1876.

Historical Accounts

Let us listen to the stories of some of Doctor Morton's patients:

Case I. Mrs. J. the mother of three, was hiking in 1868, when

"Descending a steep ravine, I trod upon quite a large stone which rolled from under my foot, causing me to slip, throwing my entire weight upon the forward foot…the pain was intense and accompanied by fainting sensations…I walked to the nearest valley…where for hours I endured great suffering. After this I found it impossible to wear a shoe even for a few moments, the least pressure inducing an attack of severe pain. At no time did the foot or toe swell or present any evidence of having been injured. During the [next] five years the foot was never entirely free from pain, often my suffering has been very severe coming on in paroxysms. I have been able only to wear a very large shoe, and only for a limited space of time, ..being obliged to remove it every half hour or so, to relieve the foot. Even at night I have suffered intensely; slight pressure of the finger on the tender spot [4TH toe, near the bone of the foot] causes the same sensation as wearing a shoe. During the past year or so I have walked but little, and have consequently suffered much less."

Case VII. Mrs. C.H.K. of Philadelphia, age 53, wrote

"The queer feeling, which has been in my left foot for 30 years, is a painful condition. The pain is in and about the joint of the fourth toe, with occasional attacks of intense suffering, when the pain extends to the knee, and if my shoe is not instantly removed with the attack comes on, the pain reaches the hip…it seems that the least pressure will produce the same result. Often my sufferings have been exceedingly acute, and coming on without any warning…My eldest sister has been similarly affected still longer than myself, but in her right foot, the same toe and joint…Two of my friends suffer in like manner at the present time. In one, the pain is relieved by placing the foot on the ground with the shoe off, and thus spreading the toes."

Case X. Mrs. R, 28 years old, of New York. Consult date 10/14/1875

"Some 10 or 12 years ago, while skating, I injured my left foot. It was thought that I ruptured a tendon, but that was not confirmed. My sufferings were very acute , and I was confined a long time to my room. After this, neuralgic attacks came on, sometimes at night without cause. I have always referred the pain to the joint of the fourth toe. For many years I have carried about me a vial of chloroform, the only application which has ever relieved the pain, and this is now losing its effect."

Examination of specimens removed by Morton (the three joints, one toe and nerves next to the joints) found only normal structures.

The Senator and State Police

Doctor S. (not his real name) worked at the same hospital that I did, and therefore knew of my interest in nerves.

Children's Hospital was begun in 1909 by the Johns Hopkins Hospital's Orthopedic Surgeons and a Plastic Surgeon as a place, in a country like setting, to care for children with bone infections and polio. Children's Hospital transitioned into a hospital for adults and children cared for by Orthopedic and Plastic Surgeons. The residents from Johns Hopkins Hospital continued to work there until about 1993. As a medical student at Johns Hopkins School of Medicine, I first watched Doctor Raymond M. Curtis do hand surgery there, on Tuesdays, in the summer of 1968. At the time Doctor S. had this conversation with me, I was doing Hand Surgery in room 2, at Children's Hospital, the same room in which Doctor Curtis, who inspired me to study nerves in the hand, used to operate. Doctor Curtis retired in May, 1982.

Doctor S. is an excellent Orthopedic Surgeon. One day in the operating room, in 1988, he told me about a perplexing patient.

"Lee," he said calling me over to him, " I see you doing all these nerve operations on hands, and now you have begun to do them on feet. Unusual for a Plastic Surgeon."

"Yes," I said, not knowing where this conversation was going, and thinking that this conservative Orthopedic surgeon was going to tell me a Plastic Surgeon should not be operating on nerves in the feet!

"Lee," he continued in that Professorial way that comes with having trained at one of the United States's premiere medical institutions, "I am caring for a member of The Legislature. This person has had two years of intense pain, sudden onset. When the attacks occur, they are of sufficient pain in the foot to make him collapse on the floor of Congresss. He has to rip his shoe off. The State Troopers bring him to me in Baltimore by car. The pain is in different toes, sometimes the second, sometimes the third, and sometimes the fourth. Sometimes the right, sometimes the left foot. The pain responds to cortisone injections. x-rays are normal. This person used to be a terrific athlete, tennis, squash, and now golf. But this is crippling him."

"What can I do to help," I asked.

Doctor S. continued, "Lee. It seems like the diagnosis should be a Morton's neuroma. But that occurs typically in the 4TH toe, and is not often bilateral. I would not like to be taking several nerves out of each foot for this man. Lee, you are a good diagnostician. Would you see him for me?"

"Sure, I would. But I am going to have to learn a little more about Morton's neuroma. As a Plastic Surgeon, I have not even heard of this diagnosis before," I replied honestly.

Barber or Surgeon? What's in a Name?

In the middle ages, Surgeons weren't doctors of medicine. They were barbers. They cut your hair and shaved your beard. They were good with knives. The smart, well-educated, men became apprenticed, studied with a great medical doctor, and became Physicians. Physicians did not operate. They thought a lot. They applied leaches and gave powders and potions.

Barbers operated. They were good with their hands.

In England today, a Surgeons still are not addressed as "Doctor," but rather as "Mister." If I were in England, I would be addressed as Mister

Dellon. I am good with my hands, but I can think as well. And today surgeons do begin by going to medical school. For me, after going to Johns Hopkins University for medical school, I spent *eight more years* studying. I like to study. I still study. I like to teach, too. I am teaching you now.

Historically, Surgeons gave names to clinical problems that reflected the cause of the problem, and the Surgeon knew then what operation to do. It was pretty simple. If you had a rotten tooth, the barber/surgeon took a pliers and pulled out your tooth. If you had a bladder stone, the barber/surgeon took a knife, made a cut between your legs, and pulled out the stone. Gangrene in your toes? He would cut off your toes. Use a saw. (see Chapter 8 on Phantom Pain). Today, is it any different? Appendicitis, appendectomy. Cholecystitis (gall bladder problem), cholecystectomy (remove gall bladder).

A "neuroma" (as you will read in Chapter 1) is a collection of nerve endings that grow from an injured nerve into a small round lump. Often this neuroma is painful, especially if it is on the end of a sensory nerve that is attached to a moving part or is touched. The pain can be intense.

So what should a surgeon do for a condition called a Morton's neuroma? Remove the nerve. Logically the correct answer, but what if a Morton's neuroma is not a neuroma? What if someone gave this condition the wrong name? *After all, Morton thought the problem was due to a joint, not a nerve. Morton called it "metatarsalgia." Morton removed the joint.*

Prior to 1956, the condition in which someone has problems from the neck and shoulder down to their fingers, with aching, numbness, weakness, and coldness in their hand, was called the Scalenus Anticus Syndrome (see Chapter 5) The anterior scalene is a muscle. What did surgeons do for this? They removed the muscle. Correct name, correct operation. However, in 1956 the name for this condition changed. A Physical Therapist named Peet (correct name), from the Mayo Clinic, wrote an important paper. The paper had great exercises to do to stretch the scalenus anticus and strengthen other muscles. The title of Peet's paper was "Thoracic Outlet Syndrome." He correctly said that compression occurs to nerves (brachial plexus) that cross over the ribs from the neck as the travel to the arm. The thoracic outlet has a rib associated with it. Now what do you think became the next most popular way to treat the former Scalenus Anticus Syndrome? You guessed it: Removal of a rib! If this condition were named "Brachial Plexus Compression in the Thoracic Inlet" (The thoracic outlet is really the diaphragm; the thoracic inlet is the neck.), the correct treatment for this *nerve compression* would be realized again, which is to decompress the nerves by removing the muscle.

What if Morton's neuroma were really a nerve compression?

If Morton's neuroma were a nerve compression, the problem would be called Compression of the Interdigital Nerve. The surgeon, or even a barber, would know what to do. Decompress the nerve!

Having a Ball Doing Research

Many patients with Morton's neuroma symptoms complain that they are stepping on a marble, or that there is small pebble in the ball of their foot. "Pain shoots into my toe when I step hard on the ball of my foot."

When William Steward Halsted, MD, began the Department of Surgery at Johns Hopkins University School of Medicine in 1889. He taught, among so many other important educational concepts, that the surgeon should take puzzling patient problems into the laboratory to solve. Find a solution, and bring it back to heal the patient. In this way, he followed in the footsteps of the founder of scientific surgery, Mister John Hunter of England.

The "laboratory" for the puzzle of Morton's neuroma was the basic anatomy of the foot. When a patient describes the pain of a Morton's neuroma, they often say it feels as if there is a small pebble or grape in the ball of their foot, near the toes. In Figure 6-2 you see me studying "gross" anatomy of the ball of the foot, resembling what the patient imagines is actually inside their foot.

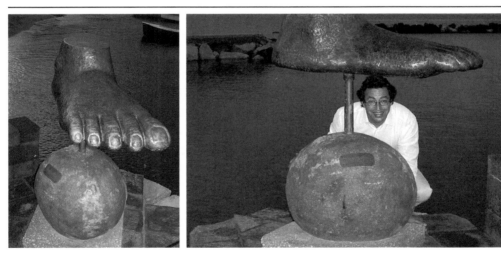

Figure 6-2. Having a ball on the Island of Ischia in Italy. Stature is entitled in Latin, CURSUS VITAE, meaning, I suppose, that foot pain is the curse of life. This is surely the case to the patient whose Morton's neuroma feels like a stone in the ball of the foot.

In the 1940's and 1950's, Pathologists began to examine the nerves removed by the foot and ankle surgeons. They found that the swelling in the nerve was *not a true neuroma, but was consistent with chronic nerve compression and scarring of the nerve.* When I found this information, I realized that Morton's neuroma represented compression of the nerve that went between the metatarsal heads (bones) of two toes. No where else in the human body did a surgeon remove a nerve for chronic compression.

The Man from Congress referred by Dr S. was to become the first patient I operated on for Morton's neuroma. Ultimately, I released three interdigital nerve compressions in each foot for (see Figure 6-3). I reported the results of my operation for nerve decompression in 1992.*

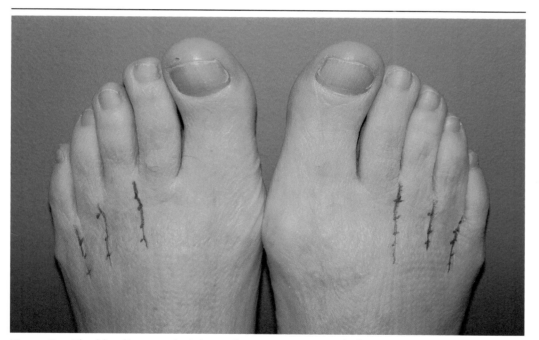

Figure 6-3. The blue lines are incisions where 3 nerves in each foot were released. This photo is taken 12 years after the Congressman's surgeries, when the patient returned to see me with a problem in his hand. His feet were great. He could play golf without pain.

*Dellon AL: Treatment of Morton's neuroma as a nerve compression: The role for neurolysis. Journal American Podiatric Medical Association 82:399-402, 1992.

Interdigital Nerve Compression

"So what is really causing my nerves to be compressed," ask the new patients with interdigital nerve compression (what used to be called Morton's neuroma). There were no good anatomical drawings to explain this problem to patients, so I asked Ruth Homber, who completed her training in Medical Illustration at Johns Hopkins University, to help me. Figure 6-4 is her drawing of this problem. Her clear illustrations are on the Dellon Institutes for Peripheral Nerve Surgery® website (Dellon.com) and throughout *Pain Solutions*.

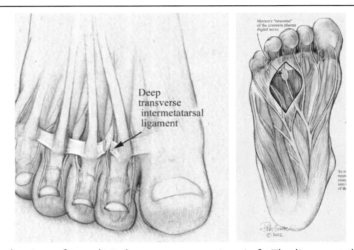

Figure 6-4. Mechanism of interdigital nerve compression. Left: The ligament that connects the toes, bone to bone (intermetatarsal ligament joins the metatarsal heads) acts as a point across which the (yellow) interdigital nerve must stretch during walking. The nerve becomes swollen, and can feel as if there is a pebble in the ball of the foot between the toes. The operation that I described divides this ligament (arrow) and *does not remove the nerve*. The nerve is decompressed, and stops hurting. Right: typical pattern of nerves on the bottom of the foot going to the toes. Note that often two nerves join to form the single nerve to the webspace between the 3rd and 4th toes. (from http://www.dellon.com)

"Doctor Dellon, Doctor S. referred me to you," said the Legislator, when he was first brought to see me by the Maryland State Trooper. "I hope you can help me."

"Congressman, it is an honor to meet you. Tell me about your pain."

"I have episodes of horrible shooting pain into my toes. Usually my 4TH toe, but it has happened to other toes. And it happens to both feet sometimes. I have tried all types of shoes. Sometimes the pain is so intense my leg gives out and I collapse. I have become afraid to stand up in public. It feels as if there are pebbles inside my feet. The cortisone injections helped for a while. But not anymore. Can you help me?"

"Congressman," I said. "I have been studying this problem since Doctor S. first told me about you. I think I can stop this pain by dividing the ligament that holds the toe bones close together. The bones will move a little bit farther apart. The pinched nerve should stop hurting. The swelling in the nerve that makes it seem like you have a pebble there should go away in time. I have not done this surgery before. I am sure I can do it for you. I would like to try one foot at a time, and just work on one webspace first. Your nerve will be preserved." (See Figure 6-4 to understand this.)

"Doctor Dellon, please try. When can you begin?"

I operated first one nerve in one foot, and then that same nerve in the other foot. Ultimately, I did a neurolysis of three interdigital nerves in each foot. He completed his term in Congress and then had a second term. He is now a successful lobbyist. Figure 6-3 is a twelve year follow-up of the appearance of his feet. At the time, he came back to see me for a pain problem he was having in his right *hand*.

Do You Have Morton's Neuroma? Examine Yourself.

If you think you might have compression of your interdigital nerve, you can examine your own foot as shown in Figure 6-5.

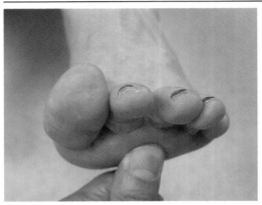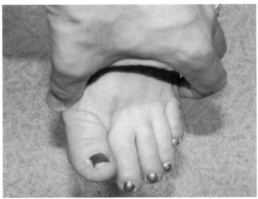

Figure 6-5. Left: Pressure between the toes where the interdigital nerve crosses the inter-metatarsal ligament causes pain. Right: Pressure of the first and fifth toes inward towards each other will cause pain and a popping sound as the swollen nerves moves against the intermetatarsal ligament (a positive Mulder's sign).

You're in Baltimore, 'Hon'

Rita was Baltimore's Best 'Hon' in 2003. Her daughter was Baltimore's Best 'Hon' in 2004. This means that you spend a lot of time in high heels looking like one of John Waters' Pink Flamingos, wearing a beehive hairdo, and not paying much attention to your feet.

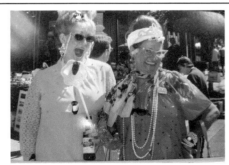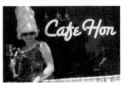

Figure 6-6. Rita carries on the proud Baltimore Hon Tradition. Her fourth toe on the right foot begins to give her severe pain. She is the first Baltimore's Best Hon to develop an interdigital nerve compression.

"Can you help me Doctor Dellon? I am having trouble wearing my Best Hon outfit anymore. Now I look a Flamingo. I have to stand on my left foot all the time, because my right 4TH toe hurts so much."

"I can help you, Rita" I said. "You can relax. Time to decompress!"

Rita's Interdigital Nerve Decompression (neurolysis)

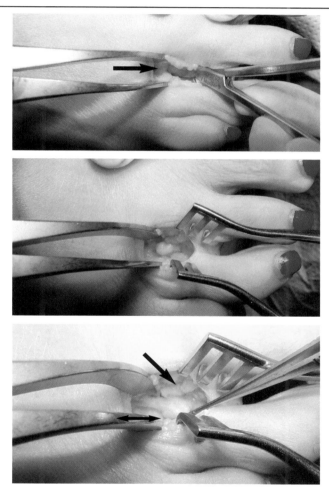

Figure 6-7. Top: Overall view of the neurolysis. The clamp is beneath the white interdigital ligament (arrow). The nerve is beneath the clamp. Center: Ligament is divided. The "pebble" in the foot is seen to be the swelling of the interdigital nerve. Bottom: The segment of the interdigital nerve that was compressed is shown as the flattened nerve (double arrow) next to the swollen segment of the nerve. Even the red blood vessel on the nerve is demonstrated to have been compressed, as the vessel abruptly stops. The divided edge of the interdigital ligament can be seen (arrow).

Decompression = Neurolysis

The nerve between any webspace in the foot can be compressed. It can happen from wearing tight cowboy boot. It can happen from getting your foot crushed. Decompression of the nerve means removing whatever structure of scar is causing the compression. It works!

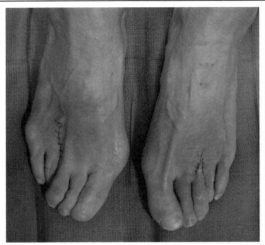 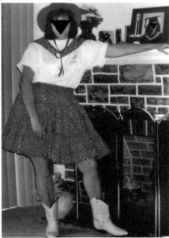

Figure 6-8. Left: Cowboy boots plus arthritic foot deformity caused bilateral interdigital nerve compressions that prevented this woman from her favorite dance activity. Right: Ten years after neurolysis, she continues country line dancing and two-stepping.

Freezing (Cryoablation) or Alcohol?

Why would anyone want to put a caustic, scar-producing alcohol solution between your toes? Why would anyone want to put a freezing metal probe between your toes? These are non-operative methods to treat this painful nerve compression. Why would you try to kill the nerve if you can save the nerve?

When alcohol is injected between the toes , where does it go? Does it go into a vein or into an artery? Will it hurt the circulation to the toes? Look at the scarring produced when this happens (see Figure 6-9). If this fails, a neurolysis or nerve resection must then be done.

When you put a cryo-probe that turns ice-cold into the foot, without knowing really where the end is going? What do you think you are doing?

Are you freezing the blood vessels too? They are right next to the nerve. (Gives new meaning to the phrase "ice flowing in your veins.")

Unless your health is too big a risk for you to have an operation, just say "no" to alcohol, or other sclerosing solutions, and to cryo-ablation. Why not just open the skin through a little incision? You can even do this through an endoscope, as described by Stephen L. Barrett, DPM, MBA. *Why not see what you are doing rather than blindly killing tissues? Just say "no" to alcohol injections an freezing (cryo-ablation).* Even if these techniques are successful in killing the nerve, the nerve is likely to grow back, giving you recurrent Morton's neuroma, which is now a true neuroma.

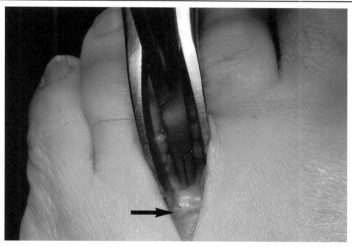

Figure 6-9. Scarring (arrow) in the interdigital space produced by alcohol injection. Pain continued, and a neurolysis had to be done anyway. Just say not to alcohol (injection)!

Recurrent Morton's Neuroma is a True Painful Neuroma

If an interdigital nerve is removed for the treatment of Morton's neuroma, the cut end of the nerve will try to grow back to the toes (regenerate). When this happens, and these nerve ends form a scar between the toes or into the skin of the bottom of the foot, a painful true neuroma will form. This is a very difficult problem to correct. The problem with walking and pain is now going to present almost all the time. This problem will require a totally different type of operation.

In 1988, I was referred a young college student who had a Morton's neuroma removed through an incision on the top of his foot. A true neuroma formed. He was unable to run on the track team. He was unable even to walk to class. As I began to think through this problem, I realized that there were no muscles large enough in the forefoot, the ball of the foot, in which to hide the end of the interdigital nerve. In the hand, I would put the end of a nerve to the finger into a bone in the finger, or into a muscle in the wrist. What was the solution for the foot? I decided to place the end of the nerve into the arch of the foot, since the arch carries on direct pressure while walking, and the nerve end would be safe there. *The first time I did this operation, I did it for that young runner.* He gave me his trophy from his first track team win. I published this case report in 1989.* This requires identifying the nerves to all the toes through the bottom of the foot (Figure 6-10).

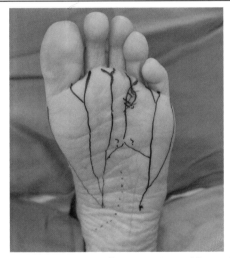

Figure 6-10. Recurrent Morton's Neuroma. When treating a Morton's neuroma by excision of the nerve fails, a true, painful neuroma forms. This pain is located (arrow) where the cut end of the nerve grows into the bottom of the foot. To correct this, the known pathway for the nerves is drawn on the bottom of the foot. Here, a branch of the medial plantar nerve (MP) and a branch of the lateral plantar (LP) will connect in the painful neuroma, similar to the anatomy of Figure 6-4. Each of these connections (marked with a ?) will need to be divided. The dotted line is the proposed incision.

*Dellon AL: Treatment of recurrent metatarsalgia by neuroma resection and muscle implantation: Case report and algorithm for management of Morton's "neuroma". Microsurgery 10:256-259, 1989.

Surgery for Failed Morton's Neuroma

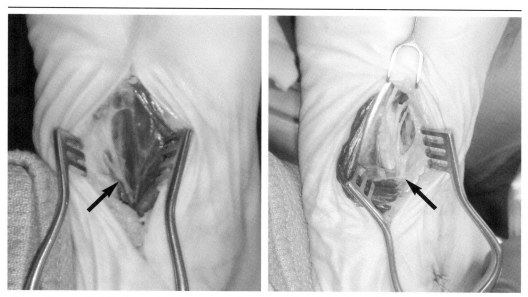

Figure 6-11. Left: The lateral plantar nerve is exposed and the branches to the 4th and 5th toe are identified (arrow). Right: The medial plantar nerve is exposed and the branches to the first three toes are identified (arrow). This is a right foot.

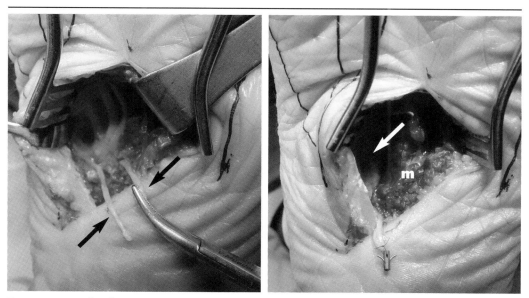

Figure 6-12. Left: The connecting nerves to the painful neuroma have been identified and divided (arrows). Right: The two nerves have been connected to a small metal "anchor" that is going to be used to suspend the nerves high in the arch of the foot (white arrow), so they cannot come back down into the weight bearing part of the foot again The nerve endings and the "anchor" will then be covered by the muscle (**m**) layers shown.

At first, I used a suture to connect the nerve into the arch. In 1998, a Plastic Surgeon working with me from Florida, David Halpern, MD, suggested I use a little metal "anchor" to secure the nerves into this area. I began doing this (Figure 6-13). It is a good technical improvement for insuring the nerve endings are safe in the new deep location.

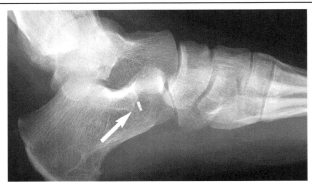

Figure 6-13. Small metal "anchor" (arrow) holding nerve ends into the arch of the foot so painful neuroma is no longer in the weight bearing part of the foot.

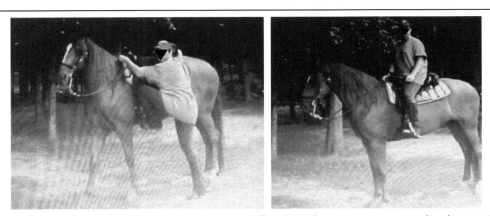

Figure 6-14. Left: Sondra S. putting her operated foot into the stirrup to mount her horse, 6 months after the surgery for her recurrent neuroma (operation shown above). Right: She wrote "Last Sunday we rode 2.5 hours, and about 2.5 hours today. Last week we had a lot of steep downhill riding and my foot hurt, but eased when the slope was reduced. Today it only hurt a little bit and it was a beautiful ride. Thank you Doctor Dellon."

Confusing Morton's Neuroma with Neuropathy or with Tarsal Tunnels Syndrome

"Doctor Dellon, I had a Morton's neuroma removed. I was better for a little while. Now the ball of my foot hurts, is numb, and it is spreading to my other foot? Can you help me?"

In Chapter 1, you will learn about neuropathy and nerve compression. In the foot, numbness of the ball of the foot, and similar feelings in both feet are NOT related to interdigital nerve compression. Sometimes, because an interdigital nerve compression gives symptoms first, your Doctor has focused on that one nerve. Now you must determine if nerves in the top and bottom of your feet are involved. *You need to have neurosensory testing with the Pressure-Specified Sensory Device™.*

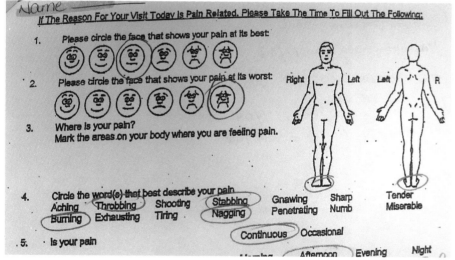

Figure 6-15. Patient who had previous surgery for Morton's Neuroma filled out this form on the day she came to see me because of complaints about failure of that operation. Note that the areas of pain are the top and bottom of both feet. This is a neuropathy pattern.

If the top of the foot has not problems, and the bottom of the foot is numb, then most likely there is compression of the tibial nerve in the tarsal tunnel. In our series of patients who have failed to get better after traditional Morton's neuroma surgery, about 75% have pressure on the tibial nerve and its branches in the four medial ankle tunnels (see Chapter 3, and Figure 6-16).

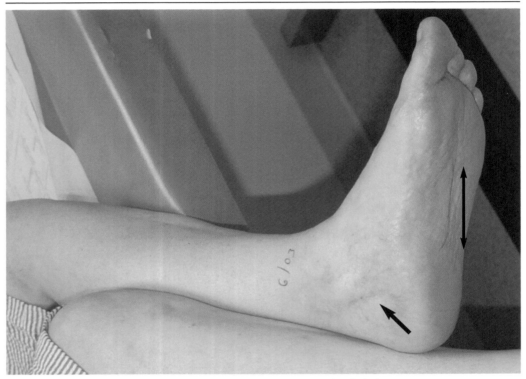

Figure 6-16. Tarsal Tunnels Syndrome present in patient with "failed" Morton's neuroma surgery. At the first surgery, this patient had the interdigital nerve removed from the top of the foot, but never got better AND a true neuroma formed. Here are scars in the patient one year after I operated to release the four medial ankle tunnels (single arrow) and move the true neuroma from the ball of the foot into the arch of the foot (double arrow).

To determine, traditional , painful, electrodiagnostic nerve conduction testing is usually NOT helpful in at least half of patients. Neurosensory testing with the Pressure-Specified Sensory Device™ is not painful and is more sensitive. This test can document nerve function (see Figure 6-17).

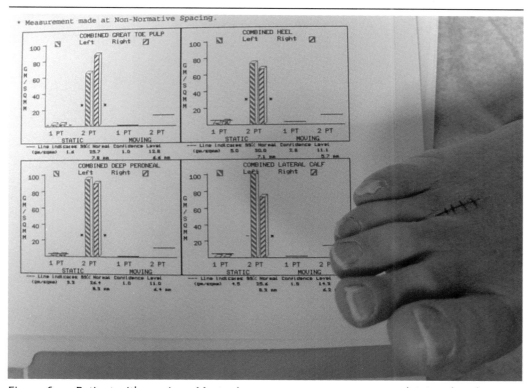

Figure 6-17. Patient with previous Morton's neuroma surgery, now complaining that the surgery failed, and that the problem is in both feet. Neurosensory testing with the Pressure-Specified Sensory Device™ (PSSD) is painless and documents what nerve problems are present. Above, note the blue (left foot) and red (right foot) have bars that are elevated, almost off the chart, for the amount of pressure required to determine whether one or two metal prongs are touching the skin. There are * (asterisks) present next to these bars, indicating nerves are dying. The nerves to the bottom of the foot (big toe and heel, the tibial nerve) are abnormal as are the nerves to the top of the foot (peroneal and calf). This is the definition of a neuropathy. This patient will be found to have either diabetes or perhaps we will never know why they have neuropathy. *Their new symptoms however are NOT due to failed Morton's neuroma surgery, but to neuropathy. Neurosensory testing with PSSD is critical for the correct diagnosis of foot pain.*

The best way to identify the presence of an underlying neuropathy from diabetes, or any source, and the best way to identify the presence of compression of the tibial nerve co-existing in the patient with symptoms of interdigital nerve compression is to *do neurosensory testing with the Pressure-Specified Sensory Device™ in each patient complaining of pain or numbness in the foot or feet.*

Pain Solutions Summary

The nerves to the toes can become pinched, compressed, or entrapped between the bones and underneath a ligament that connects the bones.

This can come from an injury or tight shoes. Often we do not know why it happens.

This interdigital nerve compression has been called a neuroma, which means a truly damaged nerve. The treatment for a neuroma is to cut out the neuroma. The treatment for a compressed nerve is to decompress it.

After traditional measures to relieve the pain of the pebble in the bottom of the foot have failed, such as less tight shoes, less step aerobics, cortisone injection, and anti-inflammatory drugs, do not have the nerve cut out. Have the nerve decompressed. Do a neurolysis, not a neurectomy.

If you cut out the nerve, a true neuroma will form. Then the bottom of the foot must be opened, and this painful neuroma relocated to the arch of the foot. This is a difficult operation, but will solve this pain problem.

Visit Dellon.com or call +1 877-DELLON-1 (+1 877-335-5661) for more information.

7

Chapter Seven
RSD: Really Stupid Diagnosis

"Under such torments the temper changes … the bravest soldier becomes a coward … in cases of burning pain … the most terrible of all tortures which a nerve wound may inflict."

Really Stupid Diagnosis

"Perhaps few persons who are not physicians can realize the influence which long-continued and unendurable pain may have on both body and mind... Under such torments the temper changes, the most amiable grow irritable, the bravest soldier becomes a coward, and the strongest man is scarcely less nervous than the most hysterical girl. Nothing can better illustrate the extent to which these statements may be true than the cases of burning pain, or, as I prefer to term it, *Causalgia*, the most terrible of all tortures which a nerve wound may inflict."

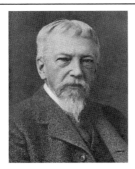

Figure 7-1. Silas Weir Mitchell, MD, Neurologist during the time of the American Civil War, wrote these quotes in his book, *Injuries of Nerves and their Consequence*, Philadelphia, 1872.

"Of the special cause which provokes it, we know nothing, except that it has sometimes followed the transfer of pathological changes from a wounded nerve to unwounded nerves, and has then been felt in their distribution, so that we do not need a direct wound to bring it about. The seat of the burning pain is very various; but it never attacks the trunk, rarely the arm or thigh, and not often the forearm or leg. Its favorite site is the foot or hand... Its intensity varies from the most trivial burning to a state of torture, which can hardly be credited, but reacts on the whole economy"

The pain that Mitchell wrote about came from injuries that were caused by musket and rifle and cannon balls. These were blunt, tearing, crushing injuries. Nerves often were not completely disrupted. There was much injury to the surrounding soft tissues. If a limb did not have to be amputated, and could be saved, the pain that resulted from these nerve injuries could be severe, tormenting, burning pain, which was usually in the pattern of the nerve that was injured. This, by definition, came to be called CAUSALGIA.

Pain, just by itself, can cause responses in the area of the pain related to nerves to the blood vessels, sweat glands, and hair follicles. The phrase, "I was so scared, my hair stood on end," reflects the sympathetic nerves' innervation of a small muscle beneath the hair follicle. When scarred, the reflex response is to make the hair "stand up." When we are cold, the sympathetic nerves make the small muscle cells in the walls of the blood vessels constrict. This is a reflex response to cold stimulation. The hand then gets cool as blood as kept within the body to maintain core temperature. The hand may turn whitish or purple, as blood flow patterns change. When we get "nervous" we sweat, reflecting the innervation of the sweat glands by the sympathetic nerves. *So when pain affects a wider area than that related to a single nerve, this area can have temperature change, color change, and sweating. This seems like a reflex response of the sympathetic nervous system to the injury.* For these reasons, pain outside the distribution of a single nerve, associated with these types of sympathetic responses was given then name REFLEX SYMPATHETIC DYSTROPHY (RSD).

The whole name thing for pain became increasingly confusing after that. Some patients did not get better when the sympathetic nerves were blocked with a local anesthetic. So around 1986, some new names arose; sympathetic-maintained and sympathetic-independent pain (SMP and SIP). Well to most patients who remained in chronic pain, SMP just meant "some more pain." And then the International Association for the Study of Pain (IASP) around 1994 decided to change the name again: Chronic Regional Pain Syndrome I or II (CRPS I or II). You should know that CRPS I = RSD and CRPS II = Causalgia. To get it straight some people now remember this by saying they have CRPS/RSD. History repeats itself? To most people who remain in chronic pain, CRPS is like "craps," you gamble on a treatment to see if it will help you or not (see http://www.IASP-Pain.org/terms-p.html).

I still like the concept of a reflex response to an injury. At some level, the injury involves a nerve. If I can figure out which nerve or nerves is sending the pain signal, then I CAN HELP RELIEVE THE PAIN BY STOPPING THE PAIN SIGNAL FROM THAT NERVE.

"RSD" means " really stupid diagnosis" because most of the time it is possible to identify the source of pain, focus on eliminating that nerve(s)'s pain signal(s), and stop the pain. Here are two examples:

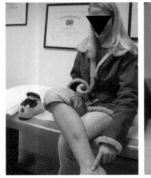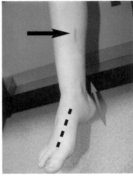

Figure 7-2. After a fall with an ankle sprain and knee dislocation when she was 15 years old, this 19 year old young woman had progressive, irreversible pain, "RSD." She received temporary help from sympathetic nerve blocks in her back. She remained on home schooling throughout high school, unable to walk very far without her pain returning and her foot swelling. Left: Smiling, one year after surgery. Right: Surgery included removal of the saphenous nerve (black arrow), neurolysis of the deep peroneal nerve (dashed line) and release of the tibial nerve and its branches (red arrow, tarsal tunnels syndrome).

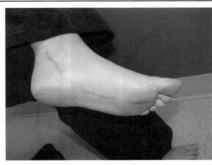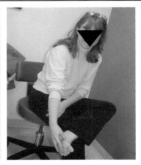

Figure 7-3. Left: After having a "Morton's Neuroma" (see chapter 6) removed, this woman developed RSD and would not allow her foot to be touched, nor could she walk. She suffered with this for three years. The incision on the bottom of her foot is where the painful neuroma was removed and the nerve implanted into the arch of her foot, while the incision near the ankle was to correct her tarsal tunnels syndrome. Right: One year after the surgery described, she is back at work, off all drugs, and walking without pain.

Definitions of Chronic Pain

It is useful to have the Reflex Sympathetic Dystrophy Syndrome Association definitions available (RSDS.org).

Complex Regional Pain Syndrome Type I (RSD)

1. The presence of an initiating noxious event, or a cause of immobilization

2. Continuing pain, allodynia, or hyperalgesia with which the pain is disproportionate to any inciting event

3. Evidence at some time of edema, changes in skin blood flow (skin color changes, skin temperature changes more than 1.1°C difference from the homologous body part), or abnormal sudomotor activity in the region of the pain

4. This diagnosis is excluded by the existence of conditions that would otherwise account for the degree of pain and dysfunction

Complex Regional Pain Syndrome Type II (Causalgia)

1. The presence of continuing pain, allodynia, or hyperalgesia after a nerve injury, not necessarily limited to the distribution of the injured nerve

2. Evidence at some time of edema, changes in skin blood flow (skin color changes, skin temperature changes more than 1.1°C difference from the homologous body part), or abnormal sudomotor activity in the region of pain

3. This diagnosis is excluded by the existence of conditions that would otherwise account for the degree of pain and dysfunction

There is no single laboratory test to diagnose RSD/CRPS. Therefore, the physician must assess and document both subjective complaints (medical history) and, if present, objective findings (physical examination), in order to support the diagnosis. There is a natural tendency to rush to the diagnosis of RSD/CRPS with minimal objective findings because early diagnosis is critical. If diagnosed early, physicians can use mobilization of the affected extremity (physical therapy) and sympathetic nerve blocks to cure or mitigate the disease. If untreated, RSD/CRPS can become extremely expensive due to permanent deformities and chronic pain. At an advanced state of the illness, patients may have significant psychosocial and psychiatric problems, they may have dependency on narcotics and may be completely incapacitated by the disease. The treatment of patients with advanced RSD is a challenging and time-consuming task.

How Common is RSD?

The Reflex Sympathetic Dystrophy Syndrome Association, on its website (RSDS.org) has these estimates of how many people have RSD:

"RSD may affect millions of people in this country. This syndrome occurs after 1 to 2% of various fractures, after 2 to 5% of peripheral nerve injuries, and 7 to 35% of prospective studies of Colles (wrist) fracture. The diagnosis is often not made early and some of the very mild cases may resolve with no treatment and others may progress through the stages and become chronic, and often debilitating."

What are the Traditional Treatments?

After your doctor recognizes that you have pain out of proportion to your injury, or are taking a different healing course after surgery, you most likely will be sent to an Anesthesia Pain Management group to receive sympathetic nerve blocks in your neck (stellate ganglion block) if the pain is in your hand, or lumbar sympathetic nerve blocks (low back) if the pain is in your foot or leg. You most likely will be given oral medication to decrease sympathetic nervous system activity. You most likely will be given non-narcotic neuropathic pain medication (which are forms of anti-seizure or anti-depressant drugs). You will be given anti-inflammatory drugs. And if the pain is still severe, you will be started on long-acting narcotics, with some narcotic given for breakthrough pain. You may require a sleeping medication. You may require narcotic patches, where the drug is absorbed through your skin. You may be moved up to narcotic lollipops (Actiq™). And then a spinal cord stimulator as in Figure 7-4 (see Chapter 10, Stimulators). For some patients an intrathecal morphine pump may be suggested to pump morphine directly into your spinal cord.

Unfortunately, more often then not, this approach creates people so drugged they cannot function. They are the walking dead. The come into my office like a zombies, carrying their x-rays, and their plastic bag of drugs. Electrical devices strapped to their belt or implanted into their body.

I believe the Dellon Institutes for Peripheral Nerve Surgery® have a better approach.

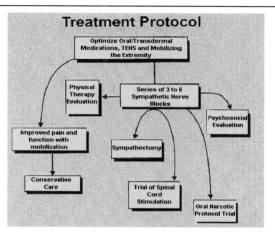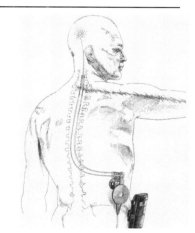

Figure 7-4. Left: Traditional Treatment Options (RSDS.org). Note that there is no option for peripheral nerve surgery. By the time patients reach me, they have been through this. Right: Representation of a spinal cord stimulator used to treat R.S.D. See Chapter 10 in PAIN Soluitons for a discussion of this pain treatment modality, and its complications. Just say "No" to this approach. The best hope for you is to find the source of the pain.

Where does the Pain Signal Start?

For your brain to perceive pain, a signal must come from somewhere. This signal enters your spinal cord relay system from a site that is where either your hand or your foot became injured. On the way to sending the pain message to your brain, an automatic response to the pain arriving at the spinal cord is a message sent to they sympathetic nervous system. This message system must go back to our origin from animals or creation from the cosmos. If an organism is going to be threatened by something that is causing pain, then the organism must prepare to defend itself (fight) or run away (flight). So a message goes out to the hands and feet to prepare them to do one or the other. Each of you has felt the "adrenalin rush" as you almost get into an accident, and your body prepares for the worst. Here is the mystery, this "fight or flight" response, in "RSD" continues to occur even after the initial threat is gone.

How about if instead of concentrating on why the usually non-painful sympathetic response now hurts, or instead of trying to stop the sympathetic response, we focus instead on stopping the pain signal itself from coming into the spinal cord. **The following cartoons illustrates this:**

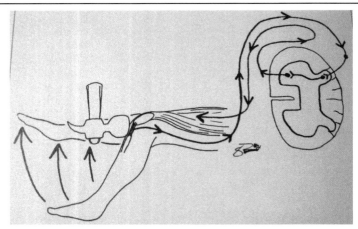

Figure 7-5. Typical reflex. Hammer strikes knee. Sensory input goes to spinal cord. Relay in spinal cord to motor neuron. Motor (muscle) response is extend the knee.

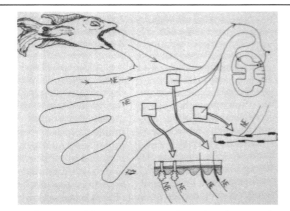

Figure 7-6. RSD pain model. A painful sensory stimulus (fish bite to thumb) sends pain message so spinal cord. Relay in spinal cord to sympathetic motor neuron. Motor output is usually non-painful to blood vessels, hair follicles, and sweat glands, where the chemical messenger norepinephrine (NE) causes the muscle to constrict blood vessel, erect hair follicles, and sebaceous glands to sweat. We might suppose that in patients with RSD this NE messenger also reaches the pain fibers and continues to send pain messages. Dellon Institutes approach is to block the pain message by removing the fish, instead of removing the sympathetic messages. Fish represents the injured nerve.

Floss and Finger RSD

Most of us do it every day. We usually use our index fingers. Floss our teeth! How could something recommended by every dentist in the world cause RSD?

Hans came to see me from Germany (not his real name or real country, but he was from Europe). Two years previously he had diligently wrapped his dental floss about his right index finger, and vigorously flossed. His gums were emaculate. *But he could not get the dental floss off his finger.* The dental floss cut into his finger. His finger turned white. Finally, after an interminable three minutes, he removed the noose from his strangulating finger. It turned pink again. But the pain never went away. His index finger shriveled at the tip, and was always cold. His skin became shiny. He had to take medication. His finger was swollen and his joint became stiff. He could not bend his finger. He began to use his middle finger instead of his index finger. His evaluation by a top Hand Surgeon confirmed he had injured his blood vessel to one side of the finger. He had arthritis. What could he do?

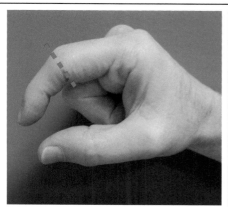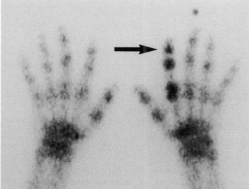

Figure 7-7. Left: Red dashed line is site at which dental floss injury occurred to the right index finger three years ago. The index finger cannot bend any more than is shown. Right: Bone scan demonstrating increased (darker black) uptake of radioactive dye indicating the increase blood flow (arrow) by which the body is responding to continuing pain message from this finger. Arteriogram demonstrated a partially closed digital artery on one side of the index finger. Increased uptake in the thumb, middle finger and wrist is suggested. This is consistent with RSD, rather than a single joint arthritis.

"Doctor Dellon, can you help me?" Hans asked.

"Yes Hans, I can help you," I replied.

"What can you do? I cannot keep taking these drugs. I cannot think straight any more. I cannot do my work!"

"Hans, there is no standard operation to do for a person with your problem. What I would suggest is that I remove the scar tissue from the nerves in your finger, and free the blood vessel from scar."

"Will my finger ever bend the same as normal again, Doctor?"

"Hans, I think I can help the pain and help the coldness in your finger by doing the neurolysis. I can help the nerve and the artery. I probably cannot reverse the arthritis and stiffness in the joint," I replied honestly.

RSD of the Hand

Beverly was 31, and came to see me with her grandmother. Beverly was not married. She worked with handicapped children. One of them closed the classroom door on her left elbow, forearm and wrist. That was four years ago. Beverly developed RSD. She had so much pain whenever she moved her wrist that they put her into a splint and told her to never bend her wrist again. That was four years ago.

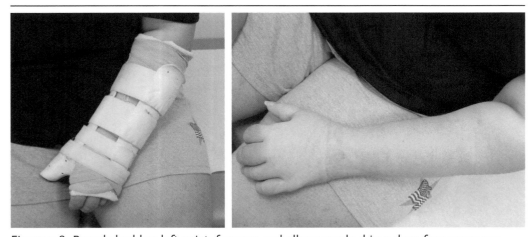

Figure 7-8. Beverly had her left wrist, forearm and elbow crushed in a door four years ago. She has been wearing a splint ever since. She does not like any part of her hand to be touched. She has horrible pain in her wrist and in her elbow. All her fingers are numb. She has RSD. She has had stellate ganglion blocks. She now has a frozen shoulder.

"Doctor Dellon," Beverly said, "Can you help me?"

"What bothers you the most Beverly? What would you like to do with that hand again?" I asked her.

"Doctor Dellon, I want to move my shoulder again so I can put my hand and arm in different positions. And I want my fingers to stop tingling. I do not care if I can't bend my wrist again. I am still teaching at the school for the handicapped. They need me. I can do that without bending my wrist, if it would just stop hurting. I cannot take all the drugs they want me to take and still teach. I love to teach, Doctor Dellon. Oh, and the scar where they did my carpal tunnel surgery hurts if it is touched. Can you help me?"

"Yes Beverly. I can help you a lot. We are going to do a test with a computer on your fingertips. It will not hurt them. It has no electric shocks. Then, I will examine your hand. After that I will know which nerves need the most help," I said.

The neurosensory testing with the Pressure-Specified Sensory Device™ demonstrated (see Figure 7-10) severe loss of function of the ulnar nerve at the elbow (cubital tunnel syndrome), the median nerve at the wrist (carpal tunnel syndrome), and the radial nerve in the forearm (radial sensory nerve entrapment). The scar where she had the previous carpal tunnel surgery was too painful to touch (see Figure 7-9). She would tolerate no movement of

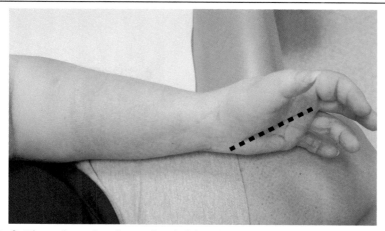

Figure 7-9. Left. The palm side of Beverly's left hand. Dashed line is the painful carpal tunnel surgery scar. Note the increased redness and swelling in her hand.

the wrist without severe pain. Her hand was clearly swollen and the fingers stiff. She was tender over the ulnar nerve at the elbow, and the radial sensory nerve in the forearm. I could actually move her shoulder, but she was extremely tender over a small bone (the coracoid) near the front of her shoulder. I knew that I could help her. It would require 3 surgeries.

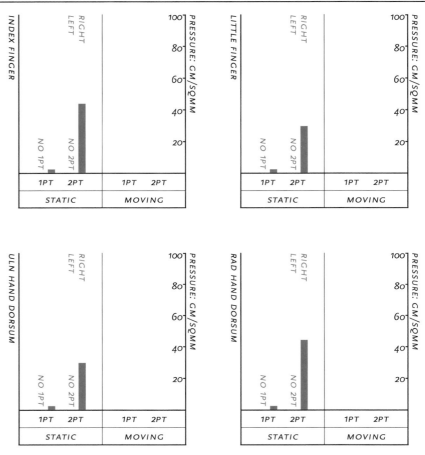

Figure 7-10. The results of her painless neurosensory testing with the Pressure-Specified Sensory Device™. The red bars represent the right hand measurements, her non-injured hand. These are slightly elevated, due to her overusing her right hand for the past four years. The blues bars represent the left , injured hand measurements. Note there are no blue bars. This means that she could not feel either one or two points touching her fingertips or the back of her hand, no matter how hard they were pressed on the left hand. This is consistent with three different compressed nerves in her arm from the crush injury. It also means pressure on all nerves as they go from the neck, beneath the collar bone, to enter the arm (see Chapter 5, Thoracic Outlet Syndrome).

"Beverly. Your shoulder had lots of x-rays, and nothing was broken or torn. But your shoulder pain is where a small nerve enters the front of the shoulder joint. I can remove that nerve and you will be able to start therapy to move your shoulder again (See chapter 3). It got stiff because you wore your sling for so long. This used to be called *Shoulder-Hand Syndrome.*"

"Beverly, the reason that the scar on your palm hurts is because a small nerve to the palmar skin is stuck in that scar. You have a neuroma of the palmar cutaneous branch of the median nerve. I can remove this at the same time as we remove the scar tissue from that median nerve again. That would be the first operation (See chapter 1)."

"Beverly, 6 weeks later, I can fuse your wrist so you do not have to wear the splint anymore, and at the same time remove the two nerves that send the wrist joint pain message to your brain (See chapter 3 again)."

"Finally, Beverly, 8 weeks later, when the bone has healed in your wrist, I will move the nerve from behind your elbow to the front of your elbow, and release the radial nerve in your forearm. The rest of your fingers will wake back up, and you will recover your strength."

"Doctor Dellon," Beverly replied, "When can we begin."

Her grandmother smiled, and cried. Beverly gave me a hug. (Beverly's smiling face and happy result can be seen in Figure 11-19.)

"Don't Amputate My Leg!"

Nurse Johnson, the Case Management person accompanying Mr. Ed to see me, was concerned. "Doctor Dellon," she explained, " I am going to speak for Mr. Ed (not his real name) as he is on so much medication it is hard for him to express himself. Mr. Ed just wants to get rid of his pain. He fell 6 years ago at work, and tore his Achilles tendon, behind his heel. He had surgery to reconstruct the torn tendon. He developed a severe pain problem. He has had 16 operations, has had two peripheral nerve stimulators. His Pain Management doctor and his Orthopedic Surgeon have recommended that he have his leg amputated. Can you help him?"

"Yes, I can help him, and save his leg too," I said.

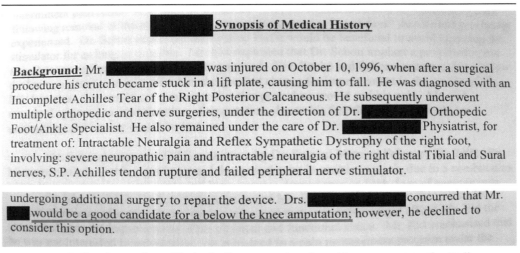

Synopsis of Medical History

Background: Mr. ████████ ███████ was injured on October 10, 1996, when after a surgical procedure his crutch became stuck in a lift plate, causing him to fall. He was diagnosed with an Incomplete Achilles Tear of the Right Posterior Calcaneous. He subsequently underwent multiple orthopedic and nerve surgeries, under the direction of Dr. ████████ Orthopedic Foot/Ankle Specialist. He also remained under the care of Dr. ████████ Physiatrist, for treatment of: Intractable Neuralgia and Reflex Sympathetic Dystrophy of the right foot, involving: severe neuropathic pain and intractable neuralgia of the right distal Tibial and Sural nerves, S.P. Achilles tendon rupture and failed peripheral nerve stimulator.

undergoing additional surgery to repair the device. Drs. ████████ concurred that Mr. ████ would be a good candidate for a below the knee amputation; however, he declined to consider this option.

Figure 7-11. Referral note from Worker's Compensation Case Management to the Dellon Institute for my evaluation. Note recommendation by previous doctors for amputation.

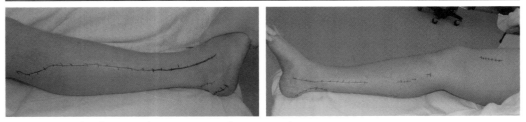

Figure 7-12. Blue lines on legs are scars from Mr. Ed's previous surgeries.

"He should not have an amputation," I said. "He has individual nerves that have been stuck in these scars causing painful neuromas. I like to begin by doing an operation that he will see immediately has helped him. The most predictable approach is to remove the damaged nerves to the outside and top of his foot and leg. Based on my examination today, the three nerves that are the source of his pain in these areas are, the sural nerve, the deep and superficial peroneal nerves. I can use two of his existing incisions to remove these three sensory nerves that are sending the pain signal. The surgery will take two hours, and he will know immediately that this pain is gone. Then, four weeks later, I can operate on the inside of his ankle to restore sensation to the bottom of his foot, and remove the nerve that is giving him heel pain. He will then need to go to detox, and to rehab. But he does not need an amputation. There is hope for him," I said.

And that is just what happened. (See Figure 11-7 to see Mr Ed's smiling face and his leg.)

Crossing Home Plate Again

Tammy liked home plate. Tammy was catcher on the state championship soft ball team. And she could hit. She could throw a runner out at second from home. She was a great base runner too.

She was just a sophomore in high school.

Being a catcher is a tough job. She had been spiked to her left foot more than once. Her legs used to go numb from squatting. Her hands had taken a pounding from the fast balls. She had sprained both ankles. Then there was the day, when she slid, trying to steal second base. Sharp shooting pain went from her ankle up her leg. She knew she had broken her ankle.

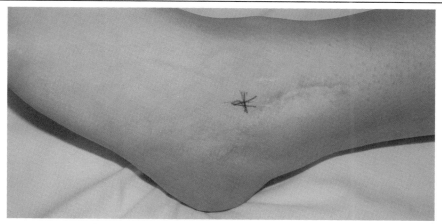

Figure 7-13. Tammy's left ankle was fractured. Note the scar used by the Orthopedic Surgeon to fix the fracture. Note the blue mark at the site of her worst pain when her foot is touched. She also has pain in her ankle when she walks. She uses a cane now or crutches. It is four years since she her injury. She is 19 years old. There is still hope for Tammy, by denervating her ankle joint and removing the painful scar neuroma.

"Doctor Dellon, I hope you can help my daughter," said Tammy's father. He had traveled from New York with his daughter to see me. "She is only 19. Here is the bag of medicines she is taking."

The bag contained the following prescriptions:

Oxycontin, 240 milligrams, three times a day

Roxycodone, 30 milligrams, eight times a day

Neurotonitn, 600 milligrams, four times a day

Topramax, 15 milligrams, once a day

Senna Max twice a day (constipation from the narcotics)

"Who referred you to see me?" I asked.

Tammy answered this time; "Doctor White in Philadelphia. (not his real name or city) He is famous for treating RSD. He has given me so many shots, and blocks in my back. I can hardly think straight from these drugs. I have typed a five page history for you because I have trouble remembering. Can you help me?" the former softball star catcher asked?

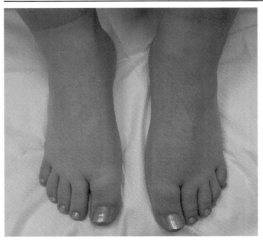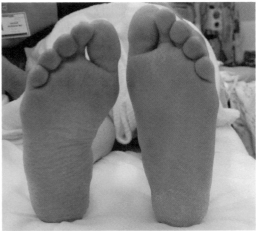

Figure 7-14. Tammy's left foot is noticeably swollen, and a slightly different color than the right foot. She has been told she has RSD. It is four years since her injury. She is addicted to drugs, and has dropped out of high school. Where is home plate?

"Yes Tammy, I can help you," I said. "What would you like to do if the pain in your left ankle were gone?"

"I would like to play catch with my father again. I would like to cross home plate again," she said, as a tear crossed her eye. Clearly depressed. "I would like my brain to work again. I want to finish high school. I want a life that is not seeing doctors and taking drugs all the time."

"Tammy, tell me where your pain is and what makes it worse?"

"Doctor Dellon, see this scar (see Figure 7-13)? Don't touch it! It is where they put in the metal screws to fix the fracture. They have even gone back and taken out the screws and it still kills me when it is touched."

"Tammy, and does it hurt when you walk? I see your still use crutches?"

"Yes, Doctor Dellon, the outside of my ankle, deep in the bones hurts every time I take a step."

"Doctor Dellon" her father, a Harvard-trained lawyer, commented, "She has three-dimensional CAT scan reconstruction of her ankle, and there are no bone chips there. She has had her ankle scoped and it still hurts. The Orthopedic Surgeon wants to fuse her ankle. She is only 19, it is too soon to decide that she will never flex her ankle again. And they cannot even assure us this will stop her pain!"

"I hear and understand the frustration you both share. Here is what we can do today to figure this out," I said.

For many years I had been working on the concept that joint pain came from the nerves to that joint. The same injury that tears the ligament from the bone also tears the small nerves. Then, even after the fracture or sprain has healed, the torn nerve, which has now healed into the scar, sends pain messages whenever that joint is moved. The difficult part of this concept is that traditional medical teaching and anatomy books do not show any nerves to joints. (See Chapter 3 for more discussion about particular joints.)

In the year 2001,* I published the first description of the nerves to the joint that was hurting Tammy, the sinus tarsi, the lateral ankle joint. In 2002,** I published the first reported patient who was relieved of this pain by removing that hurt nerve.

"Tammy, I am going to put a local anesthetic into your leg in two places. One will put the nerve to that painful ankle joint to sleep, and the other will put the nerve that is stuck in your scar to sleep. I do not have to inject the painful place itself, but up higher on your leg. If I have the correct nerves put to sleep, you will be able to stand up and walk without your crutches, right away, today. This is not a treatment. It is the way to make the correct diagnosis of which nerves are hurt. Then at surgery we remove those nerves. Do I have your permission to do the two nerve blocks?"

"Sure, go ahead," Tammy said. "Doctor White in Philadelphia has done so many blocks in my back, that I am immune to them."

I did the two blocks. Tammy got up and walked without her crutches. She walked without pain for the first time in four years!

"Doctor Dellon," Tammy said, "Can you do the surgery today?"

"Tammy, the top of your foot is now numb. It will always be numb if I take out those nerves."

"Doctor Dellon, in professional baseball, the teams are always trading players. I will trade numbness for pain any day! Let's go!"

Now it was the lawyer's turn. Cross examination began: "Doctor Dellon, we have been told that people with RSD should not have surgery. That surgery does not work. And that you should not cut a nerve. The pain will only get worse."

"Tammy, could you be in any worse pain?" I asked.

"No she replied. I am totally drugged. I don't go out. I use crutches. I have no life … I guess I could be worse if I were paralyzed. Is there a chance your surgery will make me paralyzed?"

---

*Rab M, Ebmer J, Dellon AL: Innervation of the Sinus Tarsi: Implications for treating anterolateral ankle pain. Annals Plastic Surg, 47: 500-504, 2001.

**Dellon AL: Denervation of the sinus tarsi for chronic post-traumatic lateral ankle pain. Orthopedics, 25: 849-851, 2002.

"No Tammy, I am only cutting two sensory nerves. So there is no risk of motor paralysis. Let me answer the couple of questions your dad asked, and tell you a special technique we use when we operate on someone with RSD."

"In the past," I continued, "surgeons who operated on patients with RSD did not have the understanding of nerves that we have now. The surgery that was done in the 1970's for patients with RSD did not help. The approach that I have developed, identifying the source of the pain with nerve blocks, identifying the nerves that innervate the joints, identifying where nerves can become entrapped, developing operations to denervate joints and decompress nerves have proven effective in stopping the pain input to the spinal cord in patients with RSD."

"Tammy, an approach developed for operating on the arm in patients with RSD can be applied to the surgery for the leg. You will come into the hospital the day before your surgery, and the Anesthesiologist will put a tiny catheter into your back, called an epidural, just like they do for women having a baby. This little catheter will stay in place the night before surgery, and put your sympathetic nerves and sensory nerves to sleep. You can still move your legs. The catheter will stay in the day of surgery and the day after surgery, protecting your spinal cord from feeling pain. It is removed the day after surgery, you will be able to touch your ankle without it hurting, and you will be able to walk without pain just like today."

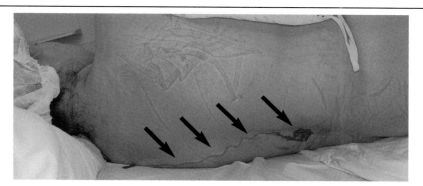

Figure 7-15. Tammy in the hospital the day before surgery. Note the epidural catheter (arrows) in place prior to surgery. The brown stain is from the iodine solution to sterilize the skin. The local anesthetic given through this catheter puts the sympathetic nerves to sleep, shielding the spine from pain messages that occur during surgery. It is a technique used when operating on someone with RSD in the legs. A catheter can be put in the armpit to do similar surgery on the hand for someone with RSD in the upper extremity.

Tammy agreed to have surgery. She came into the hospital the day before her surgery. The Anesthesiologist put in the epidural catheter. The local anesthetic, marcaine, began to put the thin sympathetic and pain nerve fibers to sleep. Her foot and leg pain went away. The swelling came out of her foot. The next morning, Tammy came to the operating room, was placed under general anesthesia, with the epidural still in place. Then I began to operate.

At surgery, just one new incision was necessary (see Figure 7-16). First the superficial peroneal nerve was found (see Figure 7-17).

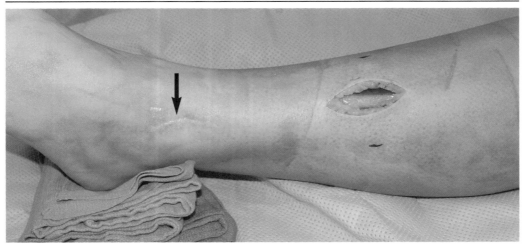

Figure 7-16. Tammy's leg in surgery. Original Orthopedic painful incision (arrow). New single incision I used to correct problems with the superficial and deep peroneal nerves.

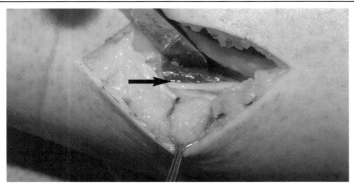

Figure 7-17. The superficial peroneal nerve is exposed in the lateral compartment of the leg (arrow). This is the nerve causing pain in the original scar used to fix the broken ankle. The red muscle within the compartment can be seen. This nerve will later be divided and buried in a nearby muscle so it cannot grow back into the painful scar.

Although anatomy books teach that this nerve is found in a compartment called the lateral compartment, it can actually be located in another compartment next to the lateral compartment, and in some people there can be a branch in each compartment. And so both compartments were opened. Tammy had the traditional pattern (75% of people do have this pattern). At the end of the surgery, this nerve was divided and implanted into a muscle to prevent a painful new neuroma from growing. (I first reported this technique for the leg in 1998.*) After identifying the superficial peroneal nerve, I continued the dissection between the muscles, working between the two leg bones, the fibula and tibia (see Figure 7-18). This is the location for the deep peroneal nerve, the nerve transmitting the pain message from the ankle joint.

I removed a section of the deep peroneal nerve so it would no longer send pain messages from the sinus tarsi when Tammy walked. I opened the

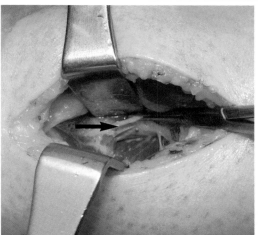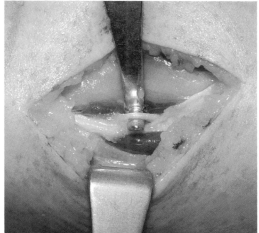

Figure 7-18. Left: The deep peroneal nerve (arrow) is located between the two bones (tibia and fibula) of the leg, and next to an artery and vein. Right: The deep peroneal nerve is elevated prior to cutting out a one inch long section. This is the nerve that sends the pain message from the sinus tarsi part of the ankle joint. Removing this nerve removes the pain message for the part of the ankle joint that was torn during Tammy's injury.

*Dellon AL, Aszmann OC: Treatment of dorsal foot neuromas by translocation of nerves into anterolateral compartment. Foot and Ankle 19:300-303, 1998.

covering of the two compartments so the muscles, shrunken from disuse and pain, could grow, bulk up, again when she began to exercise. Note there is no bleeding during the surgery because it is done with a tourniquet. The absence of bleeding allows me to find the small nerves. Tammy's surgery went smoothly and without any complications.

In the hospital, slowly the marcaine going into the epidural catheter was reduced until Tammy could feel her foot normally again. Then the Anesthesiologist removed the epidural catheter from her back.

The day following removal of the epidural catheter, tammy had no more pain when her ankle scar (see Figure 7-19) was touched. There was no pain in her ankle when she walked for the first time in her hospital room.

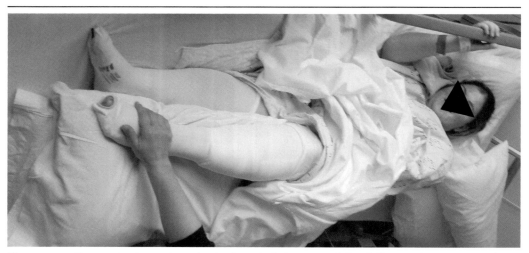

Figure 7-19. Tammy is shown here in the hospital the second day following her surgery. The epidural catheter has been removed. Note she is smiling as the previously painful ankle is being touched. Her previously painful, RSD foot is no longer painful.

As I wrote the order to discharge her from the hospital, I felt like Tammy's softball coach, standing at third base, waving her on to home.

At home, Tammy had to take the long trip to drug rehab, to detox. I began her on water walking to build her confidence in her ankle.

At three months after surgery, when Tammy came back to the office, she was walking well, and without crutches. She was almost off her narcotics.

I told her she could begin to play catch with her Dad again. She could begin to use the treadmill at the gym, and jog a little, if she wanted.

"Doctor Dellon," Tammy said, when she came back to the office for her 6 month post-op visit, "I am off all my drugs. I feel like a human being again. I am my old self. Doctor Dellon, I have enrolled in a GED course to get my high school diploma. I can concentrate on studies again. Doctor Dellon, its like you and I were on the same baseball team. You were the designated hitter. I was the base runner. You hit the home run, and I crossed home plate again. Thank you Doctor Dellon."

Pain Solutions Summary

Reflex Sympathetic Dystrophy, pain out of proportion to the injury mechanism, or a single nerve, does exist. It is the same pain regardless of whether you adopt a new name for it, like Complex Regional Pain Syndrome, or not.

The reflex concept is important to me in guiding surgical treatment for those patients who do not respond to medicines and nerve blocks.

I find the peripheral nerve that is the source of the pain. It may be a nerve cut by the original injury, or by the first surgeon. It might be a nerve compression or pain for the torn ligaments of a joint.

By using nerve blocks of peripheral nerves, the nerve sending the pain message to the spinal cord can be found. The nerve problem can be corrected either by removing the damaged nerve or decompressing it.

There is hope for you.

Visit Dellon.com or call +1 877-DELLON-1 (+1 877-335-5661).

8

Chapter Eight
Phantom Pain

"My toes are curling,
and I have cramps in the
bottom of my foot.
Am I crazy?
Doctor, you know,
I no longer have a foot!"

Phantom Pain

"It is driving me crazy," said Ted, a 32 year leg amputee.

"My toes are curling, and I have cramps in the bottom of my foot," he continued. "Am I crazy? Doctor, you know, I no longer have a foot!"

That is the essence of phantom pain. The body part is missing. The missing body part hurts. Is the pain real or imagined. To me, if you imagine the pain, you are in pain. And yet, how can the toes hurt and the foot cramp, when there are no toes and no foot.

"Doctor Dellon, if I could only stretch my toes, scratch my foot…" his voice trailed off in frustration, desperately seeking answers. And relief of his phantom pain.

"Ted, I can help you," I said. "I can't get you to scratch your toes again, but I know where that Phantom lives, and you and I can visit the place together," I said.

"Where does the Phantom live, Doctor Dellon?"

"Ted, we have to take a trip to what the old time surgeons called the Operating Theater. I am going to get you a front row seat."

Historical Pain Approaches

These complaints have perplexed doctors since before the days of the Gladiators. The Gladiators, however, probably did not complain. Galen, the most famous doctor of his time (200 years AD), began his work as a physician to the Gladiators. He became famous for his anatomy dissections!

Pain Management for much of history was death. Consider this quote from Ambroise Paré (1510-1590). He was the Surgeon to Napoleon. Paré wrote a book, *Journeys in Diverse Places,* which was translated and published in the Harvard Classics. Battle of Turin in 1537: Paré wrote,

"I entered into a stable, thinking to lodge my own and my man's horse, and found four dead soldiers, and three propped against the wall, their features all changed, and they neither saw, heard ,nor spake, and their clothes were still smouldeing where the gun-powder had burned them. As I was looking at them with pity, there came an old soldier who asked me if there were any way to cure them . I said no. And then he went up to them and cut their throats, gently and without ill will toward them. Seeing this great cruelty, I told him he was a villain; he answered he prayed God, when he should be in such a plight, he might find someone to do the same for him, that he should not linger in misery."

Paré was most famous for the treatment of wounds. For example he introduced the use of sutures (ligatures) to tie of blood vessels instead of pouring boiling oil or water on to the arteries. With regard to amputation, consider his words from his notes at the Battle of Saint Quentin in 1557:

"The King begged me to stop at La Fere with him to dress a very great number of wounded who had retreated there after the battle. Their wounds were very putrid, and full of worms, with gangrene, and corruption; and I had to make free play with the knife to cut off what was corrupt, which was not done without amputation of arms and legs…and did all I could for them; but in spite for all my care many of them died."

Amputation and Anesthesia

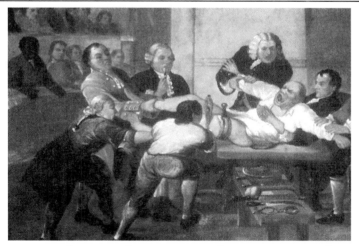

Figure 8-1. Amputation without anesthesia; "Picture of an amputation in the operating theatre of old Saint Thomas Hospital, London, around 1775". (http://www.general-anaesthesia.com/images/leg-amputation.jpg&imgrefurl=http://www.general-anaesthesia.com/images/amputation.html&h=302&w=216&sz=12&tbnid=y7ZatRabmtYJ:&tbnh=112&tbnw=80&hl=en&start=14&prev=/images%3Fq%3DAMPUTATION%2BLEG%26svnum%3D10%26hl%3Den%26lr%3D%26sa%3DG)

In the absence of anesthesia, swiftness was the mark of the best surgeon. Tourniquets were placed about the leg to minimize blood loss. The best surgeons could remove a leg in less than 30 seconds.

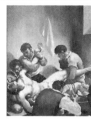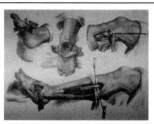

Figure 8-2. Left: Another example of amputation without anesthesia, with the patient having fainted half-way through the surgeon, who is here shown with a saw going through the bone. (from website noted in legend of Figure 8-1). Right: Artists drawing of method of amputation, here using a "chain saw" to cut the bone. (medicalantique.com)

Anesthesia was first documented for surgery in Boston, at the Massachusetts General Hospital in what is now known as the "Ether Dome." The date was October 16, 1846.

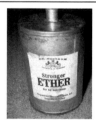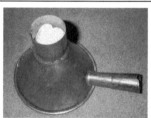

Figure 8-3. Left: Anesthesia at the time of the Civil War was given as either chloroform or ether. A canister of ether is shown here. Right: The ether was "dropped" on to a gauze sponge in the ether "cone." As the liquid evaporated, the patient breathed it in and went to sleep.

The Phantom and the Civil War

During the Civil War in America, 1861-1865, saving the injured leg during the time of the musket and cannon ball meant certain death from infection and gangrene. Amputation was the alternative to death.

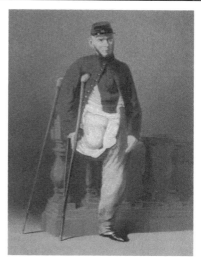

Figure 8-4. A Confederate soldier after a leg amputation during the Civil War. (From: Otis, George A. A Report on Amputationsof the Hip-Joint, in Military Surgery. Washington:Govt. Printing Office, 1867)

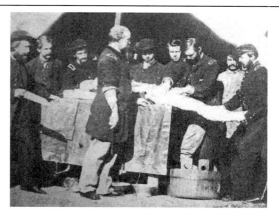

Figure 8-5. Amputation in a Field Tent at Battle of Gettysburg, July 1863. (http://images.google.com/imgres?imgurl=http://antiquescien tifica.com/photo_stereoview_Gettysburg_amputation_saw_detail.jpg&imgrefurl=http://antiq uescientifica.com/archive43.htm&h=417&w=576&sz=109&tbnid=Tq36L2LyS6UJ:&tbnh=95&tb nw=132&hl=en&start=27&prev=/images%3Fq%3DAMPUTATION%2BLEG%26start%3D20%2 6svnum%3D10%26hl%3Den%26lr%3D%26sa%3DN)

Eighty thousand (80,000) legs were amputated in the Civil War. About 24,000 of these men died afterwards from infection. Penicillin, the antibiotic, came into use about 1942, World War II. (We measure surgical progress by lessons learned in warfare. Even today!)

Amputation bone saw by Tiemann, ivory handle c. 1850

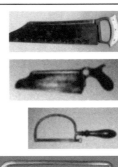

Amputation bone saw by Tiemann, gutta percha handle, c. 1880, pitting on the blade. Priced accordingly.

Metacarpel bone saw, after Benjamin Bell, c.1780

Capital bone saw and metacarpal saw by V.W. Brinkerhoff, NY

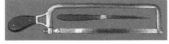

Dr. Butcher's bone saw, c. 1851

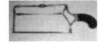

Chain saw, c. 1860, ebony handles, one detachable for attachment to a carrier needle (shown below) which would be used to thread the chain around the bone to be cut or resected. The carrier needle (dia. 2") has an "eye" in the tip for inserting a thread used to draw the chain around the bone.

Figure 8-6. The amputation saw was a major part of any amputation set. Without one, the set was seriously compromised. Saws from the Civil War era are distinctive in that the handles were non-metallic and many had a pistol grip shape. (medicalantiques.com)

The soldiers were lined up on cots awaiting leg amputation. The operating room was a tent on the farm turned battlefield. The phantom of the opera(rating theater) was well-known in the 1860's.

While many Generals of the Civil War are household names in America today, Robert E. Lee, Ulysses S. Grant, for example, one general rapidly became the most famous in battle: *General Anesthesia*. There had always been alcohol and morphine for Pain Management. Of course, we still use those methods today. General Stonewall Jackson described the use of *General Anesthesia* as an "infinite blessing" for his troops (see Figure 8-3)

The Phantom was first described by the Neurologist, Silas Weir Mitchell, MD (read more about him related to RSD in Chapter 7). In his writings after the American Civil War, in his book *Injuries of Nerves and Their Consequences* (published in 1872), Mitchell wrote his observations on injured soldiers after they had an amputation:

"*Sensory hallucination.* No history of the physiology of stumps would be complete without some account of the sensorial delusions to which persons are subject in connection with their lost limbs...Nearly every man who loses a limb carries about with him a constant or inconstant phantom of the missing member, a sensory ghost of that much of himself, and sometimes a most inconvenient presence, faintly felt at time, but ready to be called up to his perception by a blow, a touch, or a change of wind."

Early Attempts to Remove the Phantom

After the Civil War, surgeons tried to use local anesthesia and then amputation to treat Phantom Pain. They were largely not successful in this approach.

During World War I, a French Surgeon, Rene Leriche, MD, became interested in pain and the role of the sympathetic nervous system. He thought the purplish color and coldness that he would see in painful hands and legs was related to the sympathetic nerves constricting blood vessels in response to pain. In 1937 he published his book, *La Chirurgie de la Douleur, The Surgery of Pain.*

He wrote, "re-amputation should be avoided...and there should be no resection of the neuroma. I have had under my care more than thirty cases of amputation in which neurectomies had been done: none of them had been cured."

In contrast to that view, my research has shown, and as you have learned from Chapter 1 and 3, it is "oκ to lose your nerve," providing one selects the correct nerve and buries it in a muscle.

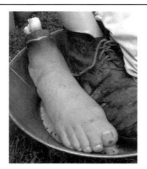

Figure 8-7. Modern Warfare. Land Mines. The Phantom lives on. (http://www.istockphoto.com/file_thumbview_approve/139747/2/istockphoto_139747_foot_amputated.jpg)

Where does the Phantom Live?

The location of the pain signal after amputation must be located within the amputation site, within the endings of the amputated nerves. Those nerves are within the scar, next to bone, and next to the arteries in the amputation stump. And that is where the Phantom lives.

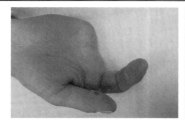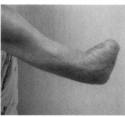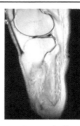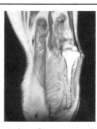

Figure 8-8. Amputation stumps are where the phantom lives. From left to right: fingers, a left forearm, knee stumps.

"How can you help me Doctor Dellon?" Ted continued.

Help for Phantom Pain is just not that complicated to understand:

1. An amputation cuts the nerve to the part that has been amputated.

2. The nerve end that has been cut, tries to grow back to that part.

3. Since the part is missing, the nerve attaches to something.

4. If that nerve attaches to the skin or the bone or a joint, then when the skin, the bone, or the joint move, the nerve is pulled, a message from the missing part is sent to the brain and THE PHANTOM APPEARS.

5. If the nerve attaches next to an artery, and the large nerves are usually next to important arteries, then every time the heart beats, the nerve is stimulated, and this can make THE PHANTOM APPEAR.

6. If the nerve is located next to where the artificial limb (prosthesis) fits, then, this too will make THE PHANTOM APPEAR.

"Ted," I said, "to help you, I just have to move the end of the nerve! Give the nerve a new home, and the phantom pain will disappear."

Diabetic Amputees

There were about 90,000 amputations in diabetics in 2005 in the USA.

Diabetics get neuropathy. Diabetics lose the feeling in the toes and feet. Then they get infections, ulcers, and amputations.

This problem has been considered progressive and irreversible.

(To learn how I have changed the natural history of diabetic neuropathy , read about nerve decompression and restoration of sensation, relief of pain, and prevention of ulcers and amputations, in Chapter 2 of *Pain Solutions*.)

Diabetic amputations at the leg or thigh level can have Phantoms.

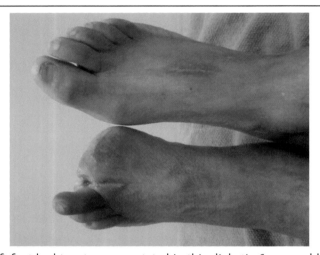

Figure 8-9. The left foot had two toes amputated in this diabetic 60 year old man. There is no feeling in the left foot, which is why it became ulcerated. He will not get phantom pain. No sensation, no phantom. An ulceration and infection are still present and can be seen next to the remaining 3rd toe. In contrast, the right foot had nerve decompression with the Dellon approach 7 years earlier. This right foot recovered sensation, and did not develop an ulceration. (See Chapter 2 to learn about this.)

Sports After Amputation

Belinda R. (not her real name), from New Jersey, loved sports. Her favorites were golf in the summer and skiing in the winter.

When Belinda was 30 years old she was in a car accident. Her left leg was crushed and broken in many places. She was told she needed an amputation. Belinda is a fighter. She refused. "Save my leg," she said.

Three years and 13 operations later she reluctantly agreed. "Amputate," she told her surgeon.

Belinda is a fighter. She wanted to play and teach golf and skiing again. She went through rehabilitation and learned to use an artificial leg, a prosthesis. She did return to golf and skiing, but the prosthesis hurt when she put it on, and hurt when she took it off. The pain was in her amputation stump. She had stump neuroma! Sometimes it hurt when she did nothing to it. Sometimes it felt like her calf hurt, sometimes like her toes hurt. The Phantom lives in stump neuromas.

Belinda went to many different Rehabilitation Centers. Saw many different men who make artificial legs (prosthetists). She tried many different types of artificial legs. Her stump continued to hurt. (also read about Dorothy, and see Figures 11-8 and 11-9).

Five years later, a Physiatrist (a doctor who specializes in rehabilitation) referred her to me. He knew of my interest in neuroma pain and my technique of placing the end of the injured nerve into muscle to make it stop sending a pain message. (see Chapter 1 of *Pain Solutions*. Learn more about neuromas and muscle.)

"That's it! That is exactly where the pain is. When you touch that part of my stump, it feels as if it is the spot of my foot that hurts," said Belinda when I examined her.

"I can fix that," I said. "We need to give that neuroma a new home."

The surgery took about one and one half hours. When Belinda awoke, she knew the phantom was gone from her stump.

"Stumped" no longer, Belinda returned to sports and sent me these:

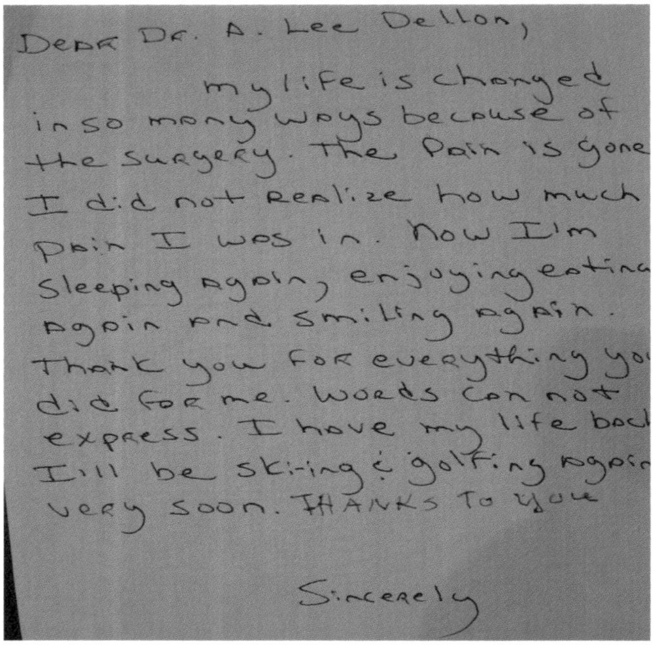

Dear Dr. A. Lee Dellon,

my life is changed in so many ways because of the surgery. The Pain is gone I did not realize how much Pain I was in. now I'm sleeping again, enjoying eating again and smiling again. Thank you for everything you did for me. Words can not express. I have my life back. I'll be skiing & golfing again very soon. THANKS To you

Sincerely

Figure 8-10. One month after the surgery, Belinda wrote me this note.

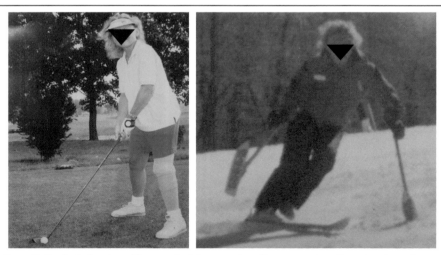

Figure 8-11. Belinda is back golfing and skiing again after removing the phantom from her left leg amputation stump. The painful neuromas were removed, and the nerves placed into muscle away from the bone and the blood vessels.

"My Nipple is Erect!"

"Is that a problem?" I asked Angela. She is 44, a school teacher, and a mother of three. Her husband is in the examining room with Angela and me.

"Doctor Dellon," she said. "I have survived breast cancer now for five years. I had my right breast reconstructed with a flap of muscle and skin from my abdomen. I have had a small bump created to look like the nipple that was cut off with my breast. I have had a tattoo placed to look like I have an areola. The Plastic Surgeon did a great job with the pigment and reconstructive surgery. My husband is very happy. I like how I look in clothes. But I do not have a nipple, Doctor Dellon. How can I feel it?"

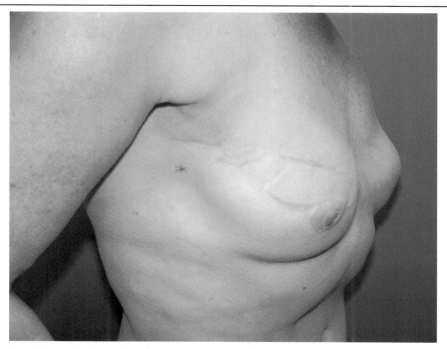

Figure 8-12. The right breast has been reconstructed by Plastic Surgery from skin and muscle from the lower abdomen (a tram flap). The nipple is created from surrounding skin. The color of the nipple and areolar is created by tattooing. But there is no sensation in this areolar/nipple complex. This patient feels as if her nipple gets erect when she walks in the freezer section of the supermarket, the same way her nipple used to do this before her breast cancer surgery. Where does this phantom of the nipple/areola complex live? Note the blue asterisk mark. This the painful divided end of the 4th intercostal nerve, the nerve that normally goes to the nipple/areola complex. It was divided during the breast cancer surgery, and is now the source of her Phantom Breast experiences.

"Angela," I said, is there a place that causes you pain when I press here, near your armpit?"

"Ouch! Yes," she said. "That spot you touched feels like it goes right out to my nipple!. How did you do that?"

"Angela," I answered, "The nerve to your original nipple and the skin around it, your areola, was cut during the removal of your breast. That nerve, called the 4th intercostal nerve, is always between these two ribs, where I touched you. When that nerve end, called a neuroma is touched, or exposed to cold, the nerve sends a message to your brain, your brain still receives the message, even though you do not have your original breast. Your brain, after a mastectomy, reacts the same way as it does to when a person has either the leg or arm amputated. The brain no longer receives messages from the breast skin or nipple. So when the end of the nerve is stimulated by something, your brain creates the image of a phantom nipple. Your brain matches that pattern of impulses to existing patterns, and matches it with the impulse profile it remembers from when you used to go shopping in the freezer isle."

"Well that makes sense. So I am not crazy."

"No Angela," I said, "You have what is called a *phantom*."

"Doctor Dellon, what should I do?"

"Angela, unless this phantom sensation is really painful to you, you do not really have to do anything. Sometimes, just understanding the basis of this phenomenon is sufficient."

"Yes, Doctor Dellon, I do feel better just understanding it. But if it continues to bother me, and I don't like my husband touching that spot, what can you do to help me?"

"Angela, if you ever want that painful spot removed, I can fix it for you.. Just let me know."

"Thank you for your hope and reassurance, Doctor Dellon."

A New Grip on Life

He was 42 when the drilling machine, the one that dug fence posts, caught the sleeve of his right shirt.

The drill, or auger as it is called, twisted violently around.

The shirt sleeve was torn off. So was Ben's hand and arm.

That was 4 years ago. Ben has been working hard in rehab. He wants to use that right arm and hand again.

Ben has tried to learn to use his left hand better, but he is now 46.

The really fancy new biomechanical, computer-driven arms cost about $25,000 or more. Ben cannot even wear the traditional, wire, shoulder-powered, harness *hook*. What is left of his forearm, the part near the elbow hurts too much to even wear the prosthesis the insurance company has provided for him.

Ben's Physiatrist, his rehab doctor in Philadelphia knows of Doctor Dellon's work with painful neuromas. Ben was referred to the Dellon Institute for Peripheral Nerve Surgery in Baltimore for help.

"Hello, Ben, I am Doctor Dellon," I introduced myself. "What can I do to help you?"

"Doctor Dellon, I am *stumped*," Ben joked about his condition.

"What do you mean Ben?" I asked.

Doctor Dellon, I want to wear my prosthesis, the one with the hook, but it just hurts so much when I put it on that I cannot wear it for long."

"Ben, I can fix that for you," I told him. "Each of these tender spots, the ones that hurt when you put on your prosthesis (see Figure 8-13), have a painful nerve. The nerve was probably stretched and torn in the original injury. I need to find those hurt nerve ends, called neuromas, and remove them, and then relocate each nerve into a muscle. When the nerve is in the muscle, it is away from denervated skin and movement, and will stop sending pain signals."

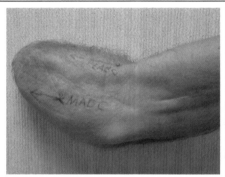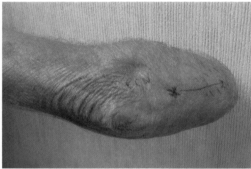

Figure 8-13. Left: The inside of Ben's right elbow. Right: The outside or back of Ben's right elbow. The little blue stars are the places where his prosthesis, his artificial arm with the hook on the end, rub and create pain. The arrows are the direction the pain goes and the letters are initials for the nerves to the skin that were cut during the amputation. They still send pain messages back to the brain when they are stimulated.

"I am ready for the surgery, Doctor Dellon. Let's go."

At surgery, I opened the skin at the site of his pain, found the neuromas (see Figures 8-14 LEFT and 8-15 LEFT), removed each neuroma, and then buried each new end of the nerve, so that when it healed, it would do so in an environment of normal muscle (Figures 8-14 RIGHT, 8-15 RIGHT).

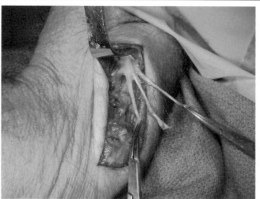 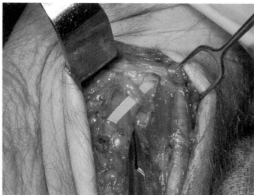

Figure 8-14. Left: The inside of the right elbow. The three nerves are all part of the medial antebrachial cutaneous nerve that was causing the pain when the prosthesis touched the spot in 8-13 (left) on the inside of the elbow, labeled MABC. Right: Note the nerve, crossing the green marker, is implanted into the red triceps muscle.

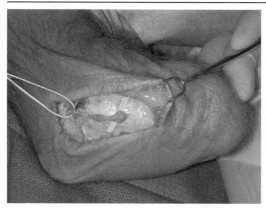 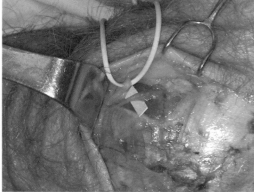

Figure 8-15. Left: is the outside or back of the right elbow. The nerve encircled with the blue loop is the posterior cutaneous nerve of the forearm. This is the nerve causing the pain when the prosthesis touched the spot in 8-13 (right) labeled PCN. Right: Note the nerve, crossing the green marker, is implanted into the red brachioradialis muscle.

The surgery took about one and one-half hours. Ben awoke without the phantom pain that was caused by the neuromas I had removed.

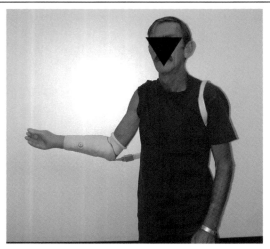

Figure 8-16. Ben, one month after his surgery. Shown wearing the shoulder harness prosthesis, with the "dress hand" attachment, instead of the hook.

Pain Solutions Summary

If an amputation occurs, either from an injury for for the treatment of a tumor, the nerves to the missing part do not die.

The nerves to the missing part try to grow back to that part.

If these nerves grow into scar, or come up against a moving bone or joint or tendon, the nerve end will form a painful neuroma.

Messages from that painful neuroma are receive in your brain as if they are still coming from the amputated part.

This creates the Phantom. Phantoms are not always painful, but they all have the same cause. Stimulation of a nerve.

The treatment is to identify the nerve that is sending the signal, and remove the painful scar (neuroma) at the end of the nerve.

That nerve must be relocated into a muscle. A technique I have proven to work successfully.

There is hope for you.

Visit Dellon.com or call +1 877 DELLON-1 (+1 877 335-5661).

9

Chapter Nine
Facial Pain

"For two years now
I feel as if there is a
hot poker sticking
into my right cheek."

Cosmetic Surgery

Was it Abbott and Costello who used to say it? One of the comedian duo teams used to have a little skit: The first one says, "My face hurts!" The second one says, "It must. It's killing me!"

Yet, as we will soon see, facial pain is no laughing matter. Especially when it occurs after cosmetic surgery.

Your expectation is to look refreshed, perhaps younger, the way you looked about ten years ago. Perhaps your eyes looked tired, and had bags. So you had your eyes "done" and a forehead "lift."

Perhaps you developed jowls, your cheeks hung down a little, your cheek bones seemed flattened. You just looked old. So you had a facelift. And maybe cheek implants.

Perhaps your nose seemed too large, or like your fathers, or simply not quite right for your face. And your chin was too small. So you had a rhinoplasty and a chin implant.

Perhaps your skin had developed fine wrinkles around your lips, and the corners of your eyes. So you added a laser treatments to the above.

And why not? You deserve it! And you could afford it.

Numbness and Burning: Cheek, Nose, Upper Lip

Brenda P. (not her real name), a 60 year old woman from Tennessee (not her real home state) speaks with a soft southern accent. She is fashionably, conservatively dressed in a suit.

Her face appears youthful. She appears to be about 45 years old. She is sitting here with a clearly older man.

Based upon the form she filled out in the waiting room, I can read that Mr. P., her husband, is a retired banker. But I have long since learned not to assume what the relationship is between any two people sitting together in my examining room. He looks like he could be her father.

Brenda appears sad, in pain, and even depressed. She is quiet.

"Good afternoon," I say cheerfully, "I am Doctor Dellon. You must be Brenda. And, I continued, turning to the man, "What is your name?"

"I am Walter, Brenda's husband," the older man replied.

"What can I do to help you today?" I continued.

"Doctor Dellon," I had a facelift about 12 years ago, by a good Plastic Surgeon in our town. He did an excellent job. I was very happy. Three years ago, I felt I was looking older and more tired again. So I had a second facelift. Walter and I went to another state, to see the most famous Plastic Surgery in our part of the country. He came very highly recommended. Of course he was a member of all the important Plastic Surgery Societies…" and then her voice trailed off and she stopped talking.

"Doctor Dellon" Walter took up the conversation for his wife, "That Plastic Surgeon simply had no explanation for my wife's pain. He told us her pain would go away. He told us he never had a patient whose lip and cheek and nose hurt after his procedure. He told us, in fact, that he was famous for this new procedure where he lifts up what he called the 'midface' by going along the surface of the bone. Can you help us?" Walter asked.

"Yes , I can help you," I answered. "Who gave you my name?"

Walter answered, "Doctor Paul Manson, the Chief of Plastic Surgery at Johns Hopkins Hospital" gave us your name. "We went to see him. He said you are pioneering techniques to treat painful nerve problems in the face. He said you and he have worked together for a long time, and we should come and see you."

"He was kind to say that," I said." Dr. Manson and I were residents together at Johns Hopkins Hospital in 1978. There has not been a good solution to the type of pain that Brenda has. I have begun to apply the same principles and measurements that have been successful in treating pain in the hands and feet to the pain problems of the face. Facial pain can be present after facial injuries, like fracture, or after tumor surgery where part of the face has to be removed, and, sadly, can be a known complication after cosmetic surgery, which is your situation."

Now it was Brenda's turn. "Doctor Dellon, I am not angry with the other Plastic Surgeon. He was successful at making me look younger again. I like him. He was very concerned. He just did not know what to do. For two years now I feel as if there is a hot poker sticking into my right cheek. My upper lip is numb and the right side of my nose burns. It feels as if my lip is swollen, but it is not. I have taken lots of different medications, and rub creams into my cheek. But this does not stop. It is present all day, every day. It hurts when I try to smile, and when I laugh. It...." Her voice trailed off again. Her frustration was clear. Tears came into her eyes. She was clearly depressed.

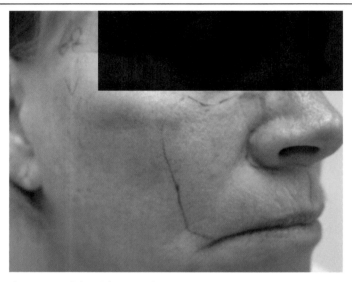

Figure 9-1. Since her second facelift, Brenda has pain and numbness in the right cheek, lip and side of her nose. This has been present for three years. The painful area is outlined in blue. A faint scar is present over her cheek (arrow), where a peripheral nerve stimulator was placed into her face to try and relieve pain (see Chapter 10, Figure 10-4).

The Trigeminal Nerve and Facial Pain

Tic douloureux (French), or trigeminal neuralgia, is the classic name for facial pain of unknown cause. This pain comes on suddenly, is intense, and occurs in one of the *three* branches of the cranial (*tri*geminal) nerve that innervates the skin of the face (Figure 9-2). The cause of this type of facial pain is central, meaning the cause is inside your facial skeleton. It is now believed by many that a small artery in the back of the brain, pulsating against the trigeminal nerve, inside the skull, causes the pain. An operation, opening the back of the skull, a craniotomy, done by a Neuro-surgeon, can relocate that artery, moving it away from the nerve, relieving the pain.

In the past, branches of the trigeminal nerve were divided, usually within the skull. This left one of the colored patterns of the face in Figure 9-2 numb. Often the pain was still not relieved.

Facial pain that occurs after an injury like a facial fracture, or after a tooth is pulled, or after a tumor is removed, *or after cosmetic surgery* must be due to an injury to a specific branch of the trigeminal nerve. These branch patterns are shown in Figure 9-3.

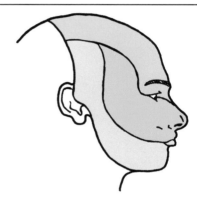

Figure 9-2. Each color represents one of the three branches of the trigeminal nerve, the nerve that sends facial sensation to the brain. Classic facial pain, tic douloureux, occurs in one of these regions. It is not a nerve injury.

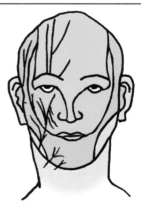

Figure 9-3. Frontal view of Figure 9-2 with branches of the trigeminal nerve shown in black. Note that each colored territory has many specific nerve branches. The specific nerves each have a name and exit the facial skeleton through small openings in the bone to reach the skin of the face. It is because of this arrangement, that these nerves are liable to be injured if the facial bones are broken, or the skin is crushed or stretched.

In the upper extremity, the ulnar nerve at the elbow (funny bone) can become compressed either by direct pressure or injury to the bone. That nerve goes to specific fingers, the little and ring finger. When the ulnar nerve is trapped at the elbow, the little and ring finger are numb. Could this happen to a branch of the trigeminal nerve? And what complaints would result?

In the hand and the foot, we measure sensory changes with the Pressure-Specified Sensory Device™. This does not hurt. It measures the pressure threshold of the skin, and how close together you can tell if its two small metal tips are touching the skin. These pressures and distances between the prongs increase when the nerve is compressed and dying. These measurements can this be done for the trigeminal nerve and the facial skin. This allows us to determine if the trigeminal nerve branch that is causing the facial pain is compressed, or is dying, or is coming back to life.

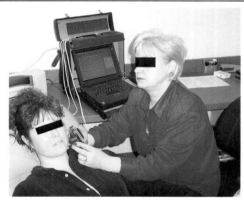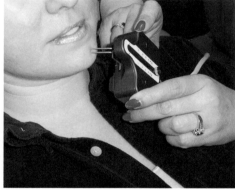

Figure 9-4. Patient being tested with the PSSD to measure sensory function of the trigeminal nerve. It identifies nerve compression or nerve injury.

Brenda's Infra-Orbital Nerve

Brenda had neurosensory testing with the Pressure-Specified Sensory Device™. This test demonstrated that the infra-orbital nerve, the nerve that comes out of the cheek bone and receives information from the upper lip and side of the nose was compressed. Nerve fibers were dying, but the nerve was still alive. Brenda knew that this was a tender spot for her when touched.

"Brenda," I discussed with her, "there is a chance that nerve can be separated from the scar tissue. Where the nerve comes out of the bone, it must be caught in scar with the other tissues that were used to pull up that "midface" part of your facelift. If this is successful, the sensation in your face can be saved and the pain relieved."

Brenda bravely replied, "That would be wonderful, Doctor Dellon. Have you ever done this before?"

"No Brenda, I have not. I have been ready to do this. Doctor Rosson, my associate here at the Dellon Institute for Peripheral Nerve Surgery in Baltimore, and I have been planning this operation for some time now. We have been waiting for the proper person who needed our help. Doctor Rosson is on the Johns Hopkins Faculty in Plastic Surgery. He and I will design this operation just for you."

Brenda came back to visit with us again. And we decided together to proceed with an operation to free the infra-orbital nerve from the cheek bone and scar tissue. We decided to use an approach through the mouth, under the upper lip in the gum. At the same time we decided to remove the peripheral nerve stimulator that had been put in previously to relieve her of her pain (see Chapter 10, Figure 10-4).

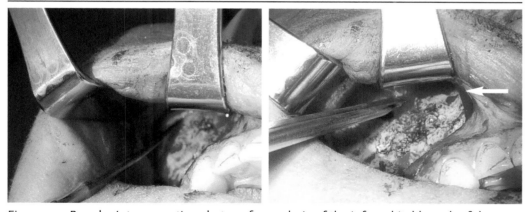

Figure 9-5. Brenda. Intra-operative photos of neurolysis of the infra-orbital branch of the trigeminal nerve. Left: The intra-oral approach, through the gum of the right upper lip. The instrument is lifting scar from the nerve. Right: The instrument points to the now shining white infra-orbital nerve (arrow) that has been freed from the scar (neurolysis).

Immediately after the surgery, Brenda had more numbness but less pain in her lip and cheek and side of her nose. She was also quite swollen.

At four weeks after surgery, Brenda was not sure if she was better or not. She had a lot of buzzing in her lip and side of her nose, but it no longer hurt when she pressed on the spot on her cheek that used to be tender.

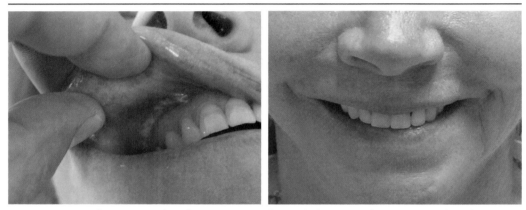

Figure 9-6 Brenda at six weeks after surgery. Left: Healed intra-oral incision. Right: She was beginning to feel like smiling again.

At eight weeks, Brenda sent me an e-mail. "Doctor Dellon, I just had my first two very good days without pain." She then shared this philosophical insight: "It is not the lack of pain that causes such outstanding relief, it's the calmness that happens, the lack of anxiety, and also the lack of fear. All these feelings contribute to the agony of a person with chronic pain. I hope this information will help both you and Doctor Rosson in your endeavor to help people in pain. Anything I can do to help others, I intend to do."

Then one day, I opened my e-mail. It was about 5AM. My usual e-mail time. It was the third week of December. It was four months since the surgery to release Brenda's infraorbital nerve from scar tissue. There was an e-mail from Brenda. It read:

"Just wanted to let you know that last Wednesday was the best day I've had since this whole thing started. I played 18 holes of golf at a beautiful course in California. The golf score was bad, but I kept saying to myself 'I feel so good, I haven't felt this good in three years.' The next day was almost as good, I went for a hike up a mountain and back down. I hope this information will help someone else."

Cheek Implants and Rhinoplasty

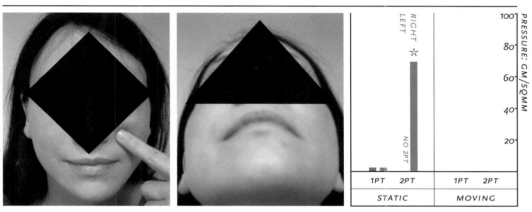

Figure 9-7. Left: After having cheek implants placed, and a rhinoplasty, this 28 year old woman lost the feeling in the upper lip on both sides, and she had pain that she could locate with one finger on the left side near her cheek bone. The cheek implants had been placed on to the cheek through an incision under the lip, like that shown in Figure 11-5. Center: appearance of cheeks and nose, demonstrating excellent cosmetic results. Right: The computer measurement with the Pressure-Specified Sensory Device™ for the upper lip. Note there is no blue (left side) bar present at all for two-point static touch, meaning the left infra-orbital nerve has most of its nerve fibers damaged. The red bar, for the right infra-orbital nerve is elevated, and has an asterisk (*) next to indicating that the right infra-orbital nerve is also damaged. *The indicated treatment for this problem is to remove both cheek implants, as they are pressing on the infra-orbital nerve.*

Lip Sync

When I was growing up, there was no fluoride in toothpaste. I visited the dentist often, had my tooth decay treated by drilling out the cavity and filling my teeth with silver and mercury. Now, when the fillings need to get replaced, or fall out, I get drilled again and my teeth capped. My teeth are an investment. My teeth are childhood memories of pain. Dentist = Pain.

"Brace yourself," you are going to the Dentist. And then, of course, there were my braces. Years of having barbed wire around my upper and lower teeth. I learned not only that our school classrooms were crowded, but "crowding" happened to teeth also. I learned that "retainers" were not just fees paid to lawyers, but were something you wore in your mouth. But I did not have pain or numbness in my lips or jaw.

Pain in your lip and jaw can happen if an Oral Surgeon or Dentist pulls out your third molar, and the root of the tooth hooks your nerve.

With cosmetic or reconstructive dentistry, you can create new teeth by putting metal posts into the bone of your jaw, and then covering the metal posts with a plastic shaped to look like real teeth. The metal posts can go deep enough to press on and injure the nerves to your lower lip, causing numbness and pain.

If new bone is needed to build up your jawbone for the metal posts, and the bone is harvested (taken) from your chin bone your lower lip can droop. Your lip will sink. That is what happened to Angela.

Angela R. (not her real name), a 44 year old woman from Ohio had slowly developed bad infections around her teeth. She slowly lost bone in the upper and lower jaw, and had trouble chewing her food. She wanted new teeth. The Oral Surgeon told her she would first need to have bone taken from another part of her body, and "grafted" on to the existing bone. If this could be done, the bone would be thick enough to put in metal posts for new teeth. The Oral Surgeon chose to take the bone from her chin.

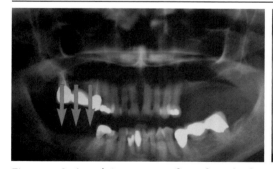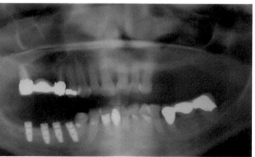

Figure 9-8. Angela's x-rays. Left: Before the bone graft to the right lower jaw. Note absence of teeth (red arrows). Right: After bone graft and metal post implantation.

"Doctor Dellon, can you help me?" asked Angela.

"Angela, tell me how your lip feels."

"Doctor Dellon, my lip feels swollen and stiff. My lip hurts, and my lip is numb, all at the same time," Angela answered. "And I can't stand to look at myself in the mirror anymore. My lips sinks down. It just hangs. I don't have enough chin bone anymore to hold it up."

When I examined her, in deed, the chin did hang down, unsupported by the bone that used to be there, the bone that was now on her right lower jawbone (mandible). She had pain directly over where the inferior alveolar nerve existed the jaw to enter the lip (See Figure 9-9, arrow). At this point it gets a new name and is called the mental nerve, the nerve to the lip and chin.

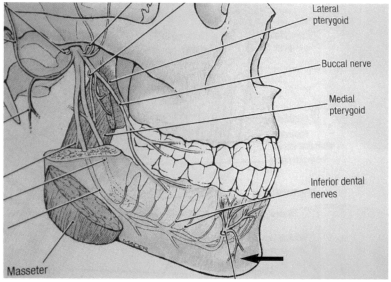

Figure 9-9. The nerves to the lower jaw and lip and chin all come from the mandibular branch of the trigeminal nerve, shown in yellow in this drawing. The closeness of the nerves to the teeth put them at risk for injury when a third molar, impacted wisdom tooth, is removed. This would cause jaw pain and create a numb lower lip. This nerve exits from the mandible at the mentum (chin), to enter the lip (arrow). This mental nerve can be injured when either a chin implant is placed to create a bigger chin, or when bone is harvested during oral surgery to create a thicker jawbone into which new teeth are placed.

"Angela, I can help you," I said. "The nerve to the lip may be just stuck in scar tissue, in which case I can get it released. But the nerve may have been damaged by the tools that harvested the bone graft. In which case I will need to put a new nerve into your lip to get sensation back again."

"That would be wonderful. Where do you get the new nerve, Doctor Dellon? They probably do not have them at Home Depot!" Angela smiled. She was relaxing, now that she new there was hope for her.

"Angela, there is a tube, made from absorbable sutures, that I helped to invent. It is called the 'Neurotube™'. I would put the end of the nerve from the bone into one end of the tube, and the end of the nerve from your lip into the other end of the tube, and your own nerve would grow across the tube, reconnect, and in about three months, you would have feeling back in your lip. Then the tube is absorbed by your body."

"Have you done this before for the lip Doctor Dellon?" Angela correctly asked. She already had complications from surgery!

"Yes Angela. The first time I did this was in 1991. That patient had their wisdom tooth removed, and had jaw pain, and a numb lip. The report was published in the Plastic Surgery literature in 1992.* Of course a piece of your own nerve could be taken from your arm or leg to accomplish, but that would leave a scar and an area of numbness.

Angela concluded the consultation with a final question: "What about my drooping chin and lip Doctor Dellon. I look like a witch."

"Angela," I replied, " I can fix that for you too. You need to replace the missing chin bone with a chin implant, and the muscle to your lip has to be repositioned at a higher level. This can be done when the nerve is fixed."

"Thank you Doctor Dellon."

---

*Crawley WA, Dellon AL: Inferior alveolar nerve reconstruction with a polyglycolic acid, bioabsorbable nerve conduit: A case report. Plast Reconstr Surg, 90:300-302, 1992.

Pain Solutions Summary

After facial or oral injury or surgery, facial pain is due to an injury of the trigeminal nerve in the face. This is not tic douloureux, which is a problem within the skull. A nerve block identifies which nerve branch is the source of pain.

It is now possible to measure your facial sensation with the Pressure-Specified Sensory Device™. This is not painful. This measurement gives information as to whether the nerve can be saved or needs to be reconstructed.

There is hope for you.

Go to Dellon.com or call +1 877-DELLON-1 (+1 877-335-5661).

10

Chapter Ten
Stimulators

"In the last 27 years, I have only referred one patient to have a stimulator."

Stimulators

Your pain has been there for more than 6 months.

Chronic pain is always there. That is its definition.

Chronic pain is now treated by Pain Management.

National campaigns to treat pain adequately have resulted in the Visual analog scale (VAS) scoring system. This gives your pain a number. Now your pain can be measured. Now results of treatment can be analyzed. Now Pain Management can best decide how to help you (see Table 10-1).

Pain Diaries are encouraged (see Table 10-2).

Table 10-1. Pain Intensity Scale (enter this number in the column "Pain scale rating.").

0	1	2	3	4	5	6	7	8	9	10
No Pain										Worst Pain Imaginable

Table 10-2. Typical entry in a pain diary.

Date	Time	Pain scale rating	Medicine and dose	Other pain relief methods	Side effects from pain medicine
June 6 (example)	8 am	6	Morphine 30 mg – every 4 hours	massage	constipation

Pain Management is given usually by Anesthesiologists and Psychiatrists. They are skilled at prescribing medicines, counseling patients, and giving nerve blocks.

Faces with smiles to frowns are everywhere, as they should be. Chronic pain, is, well, chronic, and difficult to live with (see Figure 10-1).

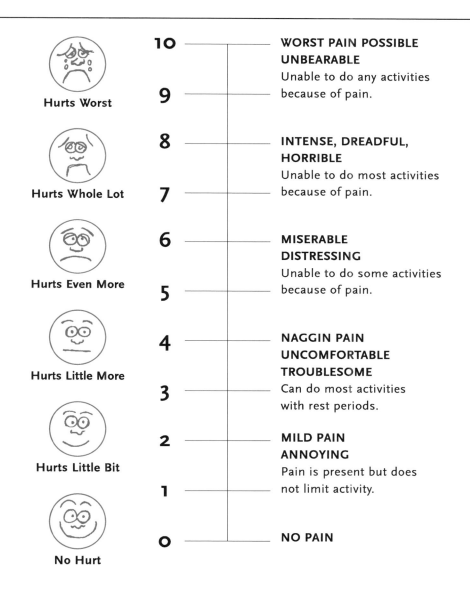

Figure 10-1. Chronic pain chart used by patients to indicate their level of discomfort.

Throughout this book you have seen the now classic drug sequence:

Non-steroidal Anti-Inflammatory Medication

Narcotic Pain Medication: Short and Long Acting

Neuropathic Pain Medication

Topical medications and patches

Narcotic Pain Patches

Pain Lollipops

Gate Keepers

In the 1970's Melzak and Wall, from McGill University in Canada, introduced and popularized the Gate Control Theory of Pain.

This theory is like the old "the squeaky wheel gets the oil."

Our brain pays attention to that part of our body yelling the loudest.

If you have a headache, and someone steps on your toe, you feel your toe hurting and not your head.

If your brain is receiving signals of pain along certain nerve fiber pathways, and you can stimulate other pathways to send more or louder information to the brain, then the brain will pay attention to that new group of nerve impulses, and not pay attention to the pain impulses.

So the theory goes.

Stimulators are the Last Resort

You still have pain. You are on all the medications your doctors and your body permit. You have some relief from your nerve blocks. What next?

Pain Management will likely suggest you have a "stimulator" placed into your body to send messages to your brain along the nerve pathways. The "stimulator" is implantable into either your spinal cord or on to a nerve outside the spinal cord, a peripheral nerve. The computer stimulator is connected by a wire to either the spinal cord or the peripheral nerve.

A Pain in the Ass

So you have decided to have a spinal cord stimulator placed to relieve your pain.

"Where would you like the stimulator placed in your body?"

"Well, I haven't thought about it much before. Where would you suggest?"

"How about in your butt?"

"Where did you say?"

"Well, not your rectum, certainly. Rather, in you buttock."

"Oh…certainly seems like a strange concept!"

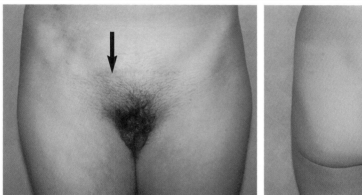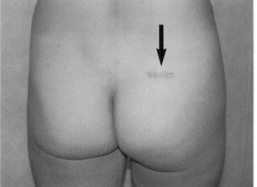

Figure 10-2. Left: Site of chronic pain (arrow). Neuroma of ilioinguinal nerve, in the scar, after gynecologic surgery. Right: Scar used to implant the spinal cord stimulator (arrow). See also Figure 10-3.

Complications from Stimulators

The most common complication is they simply do not work.

Well, their electrical function works, except when the battery has to be replaced.

Sadly, very few people in chronic pain realize a lot of pain relief from stimulators. It is not clear why, but if someone were to ask me, I would say:

"The pain generating signal itself must be removed."

DELLON INSTITUTES FOR PERIPHERAL NERVE SURGERY® DO THAT!

When pain relief is not what is hoped for from the first spinal cord location of the stimulator, the next step is to operate again, and relocate the stimulator along the spinal cord to a (hopefully) better spot.

This can be repeated a number of times. Sometimes a stimulator with only 6 points of stimulating the spinal cord. Pain Management may suggest a newer, better one , with 12 leads. Another operation.

Then there is the risk of the pocket of the stimulator becoming infected (read about James in Chapter 4, and see, Figure 4-11, the open wound created when the stimulator became infected).

Then there is the risk of infection spreading along the wire leading from the stimulator into the tissues around the spinal cord.

Then there is the risk of leakage of spinal fluid, and headaches.

Then there is the risk of infection of the spinal cord itself.

And well, if the stimulator does not work , how about implanting a morphine pump directly into the spinal cord.

Did you ask what the overall cost of the spinal cord stimulator is to the insurance company? "$50,000" all costs considered, more or less. Well worth it, I suppose, if the pain would go away. And the operations stop.

By the way, there is a cost to remove it, if it is really a pain in the ass.

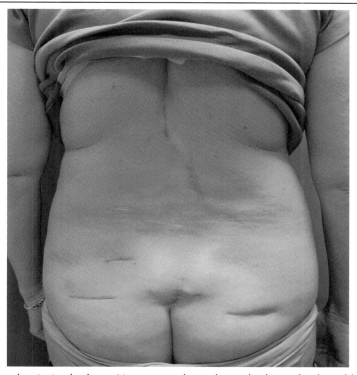

Figure 10-3. A real pain in the butt. Note scars throughout the lower back and buttock related to placement of spinal cord stimulator for treatment of groin pain. This is what happened to Janis before she learned about the Dellon Institutes for Peripheral Nerve Surgery®, where her pain was finally relieved by removing the painful nerve injured during her cardiac catheterization (see Figure 4-13).

Peripheral Nerve Stimulators

Your pain may be in an arm or leg.

Let us say that no one has been able to figure out why you have your pain in the arm or leg, but your Pain Management doctor can give you a few hours of relief if he puts local anesthesia, a nerve block, around a certain nerve. Well, it seems likely that the pain message is traveling to your brain along that nerve. Many Pain Management doctors would then refer you to the Dellon Institutes for Peripheral Nerve Surgery to remove this nerve.

At the Dellon Institutes for Peripheral Nerve Surgery® our approach is to correct the problem with that nerve. This means either a neuroma or a nerve compression can be identified, and a PAIN SOLUTION designed to help you. Most often the pain stimulator can be removed.

Many Pain Management doctors, however, unaware that PAIN SOLUTIONS are available, will suggest a peripheral nerve stimulator.

In surgery, the Pain Management doctor will find the peripheral nerve, place the stimulating electrodes around the nerve with sutures to hold it in place, and then run a wire from that nerve to the miniaturized computer that must be implanted into your body. Where will they implant the stimulator? Often into your chest, near your breast, or into a pocket created in the lower abdominal wall.

Peripheral Nerve Stimulators have the same list of complications and problems as Spinal Cord stimulators.

They have one other unique complication. *They can injure the peripheral nerve to which they are attached.* The electrical stimulation can make muscles contract uncontrollably, contorting the hand or foot into bizarre appearances. The nerve can become compressed by the stimulator causing chronic nerve compression, with its own group of pains.

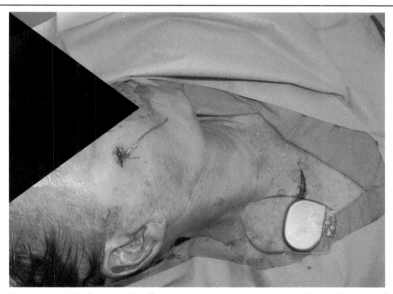

Figure 10-4. A woman with facial pain after a cosmetic surgery procedure. After her facelift, her right upper lip and cheek became painful, burning, and numb (note shaded area of symptoms. After 3 years of seeking help, and living with pain, a Neurosurgeon placed a peripheral nerve stimulator into her face. The electrode (arrow) was placed around the region of the infra-orbital nerve, the nerve that exists below the cheek bone. The wire was passed over and behind the ear, down the neck, over the collar bone, and connected to the miniaturized computer that was implanted into her chest, above her breast. At surgery, the approach designed for this woman, was to remove the nerve from scar tissue through an incision under her upper lip. The stimulator electrode was removed as was the stimulator itself, noted on her chest. The connecting wire is easily seen. (Learn more about Brenda in Chapter 9 on Facial Pain.)

A Shot in the Dark

In the last 27 years, I have only referred one patient to have a spinal cord stimulator placed.

Rhonda (not her real name) was an off-duty Baltimore policewoman who shot herself in the left leg, accidentally, with her own pistol. It was night. She was cleaning her pistol at home. There was a shot!

The bullet went through her leg, just below the knee. The bones were not injured. She had immediate pain in the top and bottom of the left foot. After her emergency care, numbness in her foot continued, and the pain nerve went away.

I operated on Rhonda three times over four years. Sensation and motor function came back to the foot. But she still had chronic pain. Her Pain Management doctor put in a peripheral nerve stimulator on her sciatic nerve, in the back of her left thigh (see Figure 10-5).

The stimulator did not help her. She remains in chronic pain, controlled with medication by Pain Management.

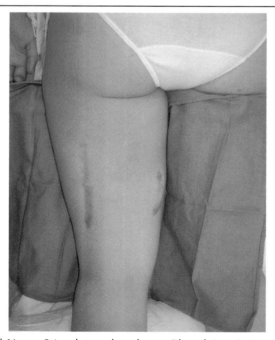

Figure 10-5. Peripheral Nerve Stimulator placed over Rhonda's sciatic nerve.

Just Say No!

In *Pain Solutions,* I try to show you that there is no easy or simple solution to treating your pain.

I suggest to you that considering surgical approaches that I have developed over the past 27 years have a published success record of identifying the source of your pain as a peripheral nerve, of choosing one of our proven procedures or designing a unique procedure for your pain relief.

It is preferable to try surgery on the peripheral nerve itself before starting down the pathway of peripheral nerve or spinal cord stimulators.

Pain Solutions Summary

Living with chronic pain can lead to desperation. Desperation can lead to desperate attempts at relief. Placing a spinal cord stimulator is a final desperate attempt. Placing a peripheral nerve stimulator is a final desperate attempt. It may be true that you will need this type of desperate treatment.

Before you place a nerve stimulator in your body to relieve pain, please consider that an injured peripheral nerve is likely to be the source of your pain.

There is hope for you. Let us try to identify the peripheral nerve that is the source of your pain.

Visit Dellon.com or call +1 877-DELLON-1 (+1 877-335-5661).

11

Chapter Eleven
Doctor Dellon

"Plastic Surgery
is problem solving.
I apply Plastic Surgical
approaches to pain."

Doctor Dellon

"Doctor Dellon," one of my patients asked, "You are a Plastic Surgeon. Why do you work on these difficult pain problems? Were you always interested in nerves?"

Often, I find myself explaining how, as a Plastic Surgeon, I am interested in Peripheral Nerve problems For example, when I teach the First Year Medical Students in their Anatomy Course, at Johns Hopkins University School of Medicine, I begin my lecture on Clinical Correlations with this question:

"Good morning. My name is Lee Dellon (my real name). I am a Plastic Surgeon. What type of surgery does a Plastic Surgeon do?" Not surprisingly, these young future doctors, among the smartest in the world (I know first hand, having had the honor to serve on the Johns Hopkins Medical School Admissions Committee for three years) rapidly spew out the popular answers: "Face lift." "Breast Augmentation." "Liposuction." "Nose Jobs." "Extreme Makeovers!" Yes these future doctors are the product of TV shows, magazines, and of how the American Society of Plastic Surgery, INC. markets my surgical subspecialty.

I am a Plastic Surgeon. It took me 8 more years of training after completing medical school at Johns Hopkins University School of Medicine (in 1970, and 4TH in my class). Two of those 8 years were spent in research at the Surgery Branch of the National Cancer Institute, at the National Institutes of Health, in Bethesda, Maryland (only five surgeons were chosen from the USA for these spots in the 1970's). In addition to General Surgery training, and a Plastic Surgery Residency, I completed a Hand Surgery Fellowship (I was the first Hand Fellow at the Raymond M. Curtis MD National Hand Center in Baltimore). I was 34 years old when I finished training.

I am now 105! (not my real age.) I have lived several life times already. Actually, four. The first, of course, is my personal life time. The remaining three life times are best understood in relationship to the Johns Hopkins University three pillars of Patient Care, Research, and Teaching. Each of these three pillars requires one dedicated lifetime. Continuing now in my life as a teacher, I would then ask medical students,

"Why am I called a PLASTIC Surgeon?"

The lecture hall became quiet. There was no obvious answer.

I hold out my hand to a student seated in front of me in the first row. "Is a Plastic Surgeon made of Plastic?" The student declines to touch my hand, as if unsure what the answer will be. "Is it because Plastic Surgeons put plastic into their patients?" Some heads nod now, perhaps seeing where this line of questions is going.

"The earliest Plastic Surgery procedures were recorded about 600 years before the birth of Christ," I tell them, "and 2000 years before polymer chemists found out that certain chemicals would take on the shape of whatever they were poured or molded into. They called those chemicals 'plastics.' The word 'plastic' comes from the Greek word 'plasticos' for shape or form. A Plastic Surgeon is one who restores the body to its original or desired shape or form." The lecture hall is again quiet.

I now show the first slide (see Figure 11-1). "What do you see?" I ask.

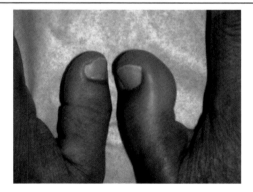

Figure 11-1. On the left hand is a thumb. What is on the right hand?

"Anthony was 40 years old when his right thumb was torn off by a machine at work. He was right handed. How can you restore the shape and function of the right hand? How would you solve this problem?" I asked the quiet group.

"To me, Plastic Surgery is problem solving. How do I as a teacher train you as a student to solve this medical problem? What do you have to know?

How creative to do you have to be to solve a problem for the first time? Or to solve it correctly the second time? Or to find a better solution to the problem in the future?" And now they were beginning to see why I became interested in Plastic Surgery and Hand Surgery.

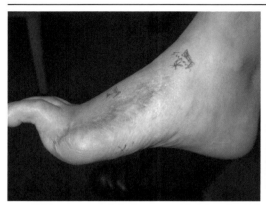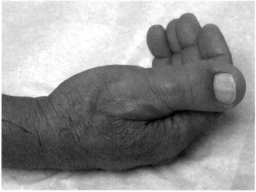

Figure 11-2. Left: The big toe has been "harvested" from the right foot and transplanted using microvascular surgery techniques to the right hand. A Toe-to-Thumb transfer. What would you call this new digit? Can it move? Does it have sensibility? Is there pain created in the foot at the big toe donor site? What toe would you transfer if this were a woman instead of a man, or if this occurred in China instead of the USA?

"We have now created a language problem. What do you call this transferred digit from the toe to the thumb position? You have a choice. You can either call it a 'Thoe or a Tumb'" I joked with the medical students. Some laughed. Most were still trying to grasp what they were just seeing. Even though the first toe to thumb transfer was done in the late 1970's when I was finishing my Plastic Surgery and Hand Surgery training, the American Society for Plastic Surgery, continues to market Plastic Surgeons as Cosmetic Surgeons. Of course Plastic Surgeons do Cosmetic Surgery. Plastic Surgeons invented Cosmetic Surgery. That was problem solving too. How can you make a long nose shorter? How can you make small breasts bigger, or large breasts smaller, or create breasts for the woman who has had a breast amputation. "Plastic" and "Reconstructive" must be words that remain connected to describe what a Plastic and Reconstructive Surgeon does. The American Society for Plastic Surgery, Inc. has become focused on Cosmetic Surgery. I am also a member of the American Society for Reconstructive Microsurgery. This society is making the public more aware of what Reconstructive surgery can do to help people (indeed, that is one of the reasons for my writing this book, now, at this time.)

"The Plastic Surgeon and the Hand Surgeon that helped this patient, four years before the patient was referred to me, did a great job of restoring form to the hand, and movement to the newly reconstructed thumb," I said as I began to explore this subject further for the medical students, "but the new thumb has no feeling in it, and the foot donor site is so painful that this worker remains disabled and out of work still."

"Doctor Dellon, Can you help me?" Anthony, the toe-to-thumb patient, asks.

"Yes, Anthony, I can help you. Let me get rid of the pain in the top of your foot first, by removing the hurt nerve endings that used to go to the top of your big toe. They are stuck in the scar. If I am successful, then at a second operation, I will remove the pain from the nerves that used to go to the end of your big toe. They are stuck to the end of the bone. And then, if you are happy with what I have done, let me get feeling into the tip of your new thumb. The nerves that used to go to the thumb, are still there, waiting to be redirected. I can do that for you," I said.

"Next slide please," I said, continuing my lecture (Figure 11-3).

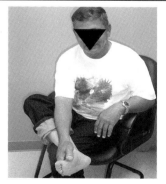

Figure 11-3. Three operations later, Anthony (not his real name), touches his new toe to the place it came from. He is smiling. His new thumb has feeling. His foot donor site no longer hurts when he touches it or when he walks.

"Three operations later, Anthony has feeling in his thumb. He can touch his foot again. He is smiling. He walks without a limp. What exactly did I do at surgery? The operations to solve these problems had not been described before."

One medical student asked, "How did you figure out what to do? When did you begin to get interested in peripheral nerve problems?"

While I was in medical school at Johns Hopkins University, Doctor Raymond M. Curtis ran the Hand Surgery Clinic and taught the Plastic Surgery Residents. My first research was in Plastic Surgery. My research involved why people who are born with a cleft palate or without a cleft palate speak they way they do. Why are they unable to lift the soft palate to block air from escaping through the nose? Well clearly if the palate were cleft, or split, there was escape of air. But there was this little muscle that lifted the soft palate, and that muscle was innervated by what nerve? (But that is another story). I loved to watch Doctor Curtis examine the hand. The hand has such complicated anatomy required to move the fingers. There were also nerves that gave the fingers the ability to sense or receive information from the world outside the body, similar to the way the eye and ears and nose permit sensations to enter the brain. And there were nerves to make the muscles work that made the fingers move and the hand function. This was the beginning of my love affair with peripheral nerves.

In the summer of 1968, Doctor Curtis gave me permission to observe him operate at Children's Hospital in Baltimore. I saw surgery on nerves for the first time. The nerves were delicate, and beautiful.

"Doctor Curtis," I asked, do you get good results from nerve surgery?"

"No, Lee, I don't. No one does," Doctor Curtis answered.

His answer was just too hard for me to accept. When I then watched him examine a hand again, I realized that the classic tests used by Hand Surgeons did not relate at all to what I had just learned in my Hopkins Neurophysiology course, taught by Vernon Mountcastle, MD. His research involved measuring the electrical activity of individual nerve fibers after stimulating the skin. I decided then to translate his teaching into practical tests a Hand Surgeon could use to determine if a nerve were regenerating after it was repaired. I also decided to develop a way to rehabilitate the injured nerve, the way muscles are strengthened through exercises or joints are stretched and splinted in therapy. And these two goals were completed by the time I graduated from medical school. These concepts are described in my first book *Evaluation of Sensibility and Re-Education of Sensation in the Hand,* published in 1981. It had three printings and is translated into Japanese.

Dr. Dellon, How do You Measure Success?

I measure success one patient at a time.

"Doctor Dellon, I am going to have to give up figure skating," Adriana said. "I have made it all the way to the Nationals. I have been training at the National Training Center in Colorado. I have seen all the famous Sports Medicine Doctors. I have tried every type of skate. But I still have pain on the top of my right foot whenever I try to jump or land one of my jumps. Can you help me?" The time frame is the year 2001.

I examined Adriana's foot. She was in college now. She was strong. She was determined. Her x-rays were normal. She did not have a stress fracture. Was she just expressing performance anxiety? Maybe she was just ready to stop competing. But if she truly had pain on the top of her foot, could I figure out which nerve was sending the pain message? And if so, could I solve her problem? *Plastic Surgery is problem solving.*

When I tapped the top of her foot, where the first and second toes joined the ankle bones, the region that is usually prominent if you have a good arch (and she did), Adriana's facial expression changed. She winced. "Did that hurt, Adriana?" I asked apologetically.

"Yes. It went down into my toes and into the bones. That is the pain I feel when I take off or land my jumps," she said.

"I can help you" I said. "There is a small sensory nerve that can be compressed against the bone by a tendon. This area clearly gets compressed by your tight shoes and laces. But that tendon can be removed. It is an operation that I described in 1990.* I cannot promise the surgery will help you skate competitively again, but the surgery should relieve your pain."

"Will there be a big scar? Do I go to sleep?" she asked.

"The scar is about one inch long. You can have twilight sleep. You can walk right after surgery. You will not need to rehab. The scar might be tender for awhile when you first lace up your skates. Then you should be fine," I reassured her.

"Okay, let's go for it!" she bravely said.

Adrianna's surgery went without any problems. She healed perfectly. And in time, resumed competitive skating (see Figure 11-4).

I consider Adriana's surgery to be a success. She is skating competitively today. The results of the surgery have been long lasting. It is four years after her surgery. Even if she were just skating for her own enjoyment, without any further pain, she would be measured a success.

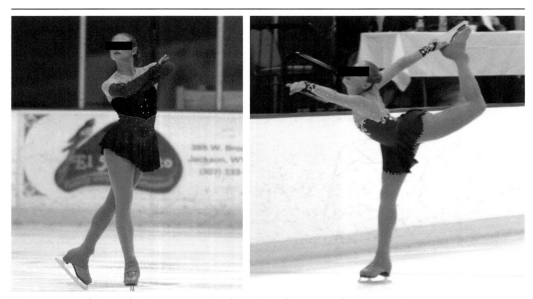

Figure 11-4. Adriana skating competitively again after nerve decompression.

*Dellon AL: Entrapment of the deep peroneal nerve on the dorsum of the foot. Foot and Ankle 11:73-80, 1990.

Keys to Success

When Adriana came to see me, she was the first figure skater that I ever examined for any nerve problem in the foot. How would I know what to do for her? I am Plastic Surgeon and trained to solve problems. Furthermore, I understood the problems that a compressed nerve could cause, because as a Hand Surgeon I had treated many people with compressed nerves.

The key to success in making a diagnosis, when so many famous Sports Medicine doctors, many of whom were Orthopedic Surgeons, had failed to make the correct diagnosis is:

1. THINK NERVE: imagine that pain can come from a nerve

2. THINK BEYOND MUSCLE, LIGAMENT AND BONE: Musculoskeletal problems have usually been solved by the time people come to see me.

3. APPLY PRINCIPLES DEVELOPED TO TREAT UPPER EXTREMITY PAIN TO LOWER EXTREMITY.

4. IF THERE IS NOT AN EXISTING OPERATION TO TREAT THIS PROBLEM, CREATE THE OPERATION.

Plastic Surgery is problem solving.

If a known site of entrapment has not been described, then go to the laboratory and learn if one exists.

If a nerve that might carry that pain message is not known, then go to the laboratory and learn if one exits.

5. BE A PATIENT ADVOCATE. BELIEVE THE PATIENT.

If you do not know the answer, find out the answer. As they say on the *X Files*, "The Truth is out there."

Problem solving for Adriana required only the simple realization that the top of the foot is like the back of the hand.

In the mid 1980's, I had become interested in a pain problem related to nerves that go to the back of the hand. In order to solve this puzzle, more than 90 dissections were done in the hands and forearms of cadavers (dead people) and in patients having surgery in this part of their arm. It became clear that one nerve, the radial sensory nerve, could become entrapped between two tendons. Indeed, there was a description of an inflammation of this nerve in the German scientific literature of 1932.* In 1986, I described a nerve entrapment that gives pain to the back of the hand, and called it radial sensory nerve entrapment in the forearm.** This can occur when something is tight about the wrist, like a wrist watch, or hand cuffs, a crush injury, or just from keeping the forearm pronated (the position I am using to type this book!). Is there a site on the top of the foot where this same thing occurs?

Remember Anthony, and the toe-to-thumb transfer? When I would do that operation myself, there was always one tendon that crossed the nerves that I need to find, the nerves that gave feeling to the back of the big toe. Why could not this same tendon cause compression in this spot? Wouldn't a tight shoe do this? Wouldn't this cause pain when figure skating? Why not!

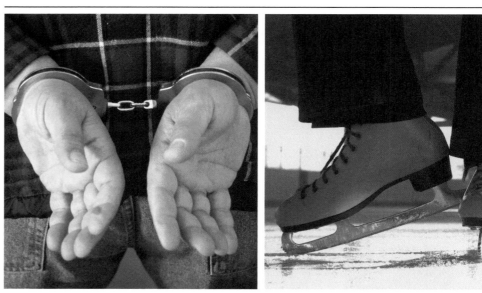

Figure 11-6. Think nerve. Problem solve. If handcuffs can entrap a nerve on the back of the forearm and cause pain, why couldn't tight skates entrap a nerve on the back of the foot and cause pain? Plastic Surgery is problem solving. That is what I do.

---

*Ehrlich W, Dellon AL, Mackinnon SE: Cheiralgia Paresthetica (entrapment of the radial sensory nerve). J Hand Surg 11A:196-198, 1986.

**Dellon AL, Mackinnon SE: Radial sensory nerve entrapment in the forearm. J Hand Surg 11A:199-205, 1986.

Why is this Man Smiling?

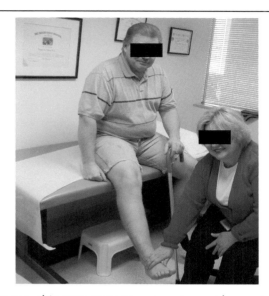

Figure 11-7. Four weeks ago, this man came to see me to avoid amputation. He had 12 operations on this right leg in the past 5 years after a leg injury. His Pain Management Specialist and his Orthopedic Surgeon both recommended amputation. He refused amputation. He was addicted to drugs, sweating, and shaking. He is shown here just 8 days after my surgery to denervate the top of his foot. His wife touches him now for the first time in five years. He is smiling. I measure success one patient at a time. He had the same operation as I did for Anthony in Figure 11-2, and 11-3. Operations designed for the hand, applied to the foot.

Pain After Amputation

It has been learned painfully that amputation is not the treatment for chronic pain (see Chapter 8, Phantom Pain). You will learn when you read Chapter 8, amputation itself, because it must cut nerves, can be a cause of chronic pain.

Remember Anthony? His toe-2-thumb transfer was an elective amputation of his big toe. Disabling foot pain resulted.

Sometimes, however, doctors must amputate to save a life. This was the situation for Dorothy (not her real name)

"Dorothy," the Orthopedic Surgeon said to Dorothy's mother, "is having pain in her legs because the x-rays have shown she has a very rare condition. She has a bone cancer in each of her legs. We have to biopsy these tumors to be sure, but by the way they look on the x-ray they are aggressive and have destroyed her bones. In the near future, she will fracture both legs just from running or if she has a slight fall."

The biopsies came back. Rare bone cancers. Osteogenic Sarcoma.

"What can we do to save her?" her mother and father said at the same time. "She is only ten years old."

"This is a deadly cancer," the Orthopedic Surgeon explained. "Most patients are dead in about 18 months because the cancer spreads to the lungs." It was 1985. They lived in the mid-west (not their real location).

"There are no cancer drugs to fight this, he continued." The tumor has already eaten through her bone in spots. It may already be too late. Amputation is her only chance to live. It is all we know to do now for her."

Both of her legs were amputated above the level of the knee.

"Doctor Dellon, can you help me?" Dorothy asked. It was 20 years after her amputations. "Over the past few years I have been having pain in my left thigh, and in my left shorter leg. I can touch the spots that hurt. My Ortho-

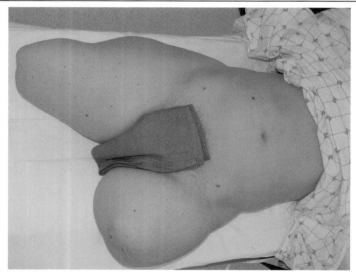

Figure 11-8. Dorothy had stump pain in her left stump and front of her hips. It is 20 years after her bilateral amputations for bilateral bone cancer of the legs. This radical surgery saved her life. Now she sought a treatment for the pain in the left stump that was disrupting her work and personal life.

pedic Surgeon thinks it is 'sciatica" from the bone pressing on the sciatic nerve related to how I sit. He though you might be able to reshape that bone," she explained clearly. She taught computer programming at a nearby college.

From my Hand Surgery work with amputation stumps in the upper extremity, and from my Plastic Surgery work with paraplegics who get "bed sores or ulcers" where they sit, I felt that I had proper training to figure out Dorothy's problem. Her examination showed a pinched nerve in her left groin (see Chapter 4) and painful neuromas related to her sciatic nerve in her stump (see Chapter 8). After examining Dorothy, I said "I can fix this for you. There is a nerve near the front of your hip that is pinched from the years of sitting with your hip flexed, and there are two painful neuromas in the stump that I can remove."

At surgery, The pain in the hip was found to be related to a pinched nerved, which could be decompressed and saved, and the stump was found to have two neuromas at the sites of her pain. One of these was attached to her sciatic nerves (see Figure 11-9). It was giving her referred sciatic pain.

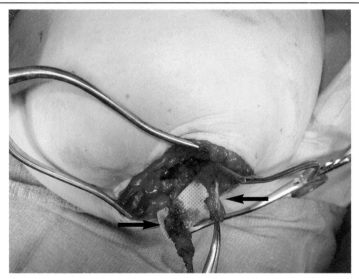

Figure 11-9. Arrows point to two neuromas that have been identified in the left leg amputation stump. These were the cause of her pain. They were removed and the nerve repositioned to lie inside muscles, so that the stump would not hurt anymore.

The approach to the nerve compression at the hip for Dorothy is an operation I described first in 1995, and then described in detail with success in most of the patients in that report. I published that paper in the Journal of the American College of Surgeons.* General Surgeons see those patients first with groin pain, usually related to hernias. Actually, this condition, described in 1874 with the Latin name, *meralgia paresthetica* (thigh pain), still remains rarely diagnosed. It is a cause of much pain from the thigh to the knee, often misdiagnosed as hip pain or back pain (an L3 disc).

PLASTIC SURGERY IS PROBLEM SOLVING.

I APPLY PLASTIC SURGICAL APPROACHES TO PAIN.

The approach to the painful neuromas, implanting them in muscle, is an approach that I worked out in the research lab in the early 1980's (read about it in Chapter 1, under Neuromas).

Dorothy healed well and went back to her fiancé and to teaching. She did not need the bone she sat on (ischial tuberosity) recontoured.

Plastic Surgery and Johns Hopkins

Plastic Surgery is not a technique. Plastic Surgery is not a set of operations. Plastic Surgery is not Cosmetic Surgery.

Plastic Surgery is an approach to solving patient problems related to form and function of the human body.

The Plastic Surgeon must be trained to operate all over the body, and therefore must be skilled in anatomy of the entire body. The textbook for that learning must be the human body itself.

When the Johns Hopkins Hospital began in 1889, there were no Plastic Surgeons on the staff. In fact, there were no Plastic Surgeons in the world. Johns Hopkins, the man, died in 1876. A business man, he donated half his estate to establish a graduate school, because, as stated in his will, to the best

---

*Lee CH, Dellon AL: Surgical management for groin pain of neural origin. J Amer Col Surg, 191:137-142, 2000

that he could determine, there would always be people who needed a higher education, an education beyond university training. He left the other half of his estate to establish a hospital, because, as stated in his will, to the best that he could determine there would always be people who were suffering. It was understood that the University would include a School of Medicine. Johns Hopkins, the man, recognized the need to relieve pain. He began to provide *Pain Solutions* in his own way.

William Steward Halsted, MD, the first Professor of Surgery and Chief of Surgery at the new Johns Hopkins Hospital, introduced the concepts of gentle handling of tissues to prevent infection (antibiotics did not come into use until World War II). This concept is employed by all Plastic Surgeons. Being gentle to tissues causes less pain. Halsted introduced the concept of local anesthesia to surgery. He used cocaine. His research led him to experiment on himself, and he became addicted to cocaine for a period of time. Plastic Surgeons use local anesthesia in the wound edges after surgery today, and patients awake without pain. When I operate, I put the local anesthetic into the nerve before it is cut, and this prevents the spinal cord from experiencing pain from the surgery I do on peripheral nerves.

Halsted, at Johns Hopkins Hospital, introduced the first surgery residency program as we know it today. In 1910, that model of surgical training became the way all doctors would be trained.

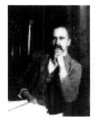 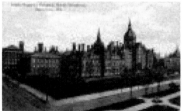 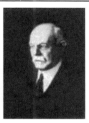

Figure 11-10. Left: William Osler, MD, the first Chief of Medicine at the Johns Hopkins Hospital (center from around 1915). Right: William Stewart Halsted, MD, the first Chief of Surgery at the Johns Hopkins Hospital.

In the Department of Medicine at the new Johns Hopkins Hospital in 1889, William Osler, MD, the first Professor and Chief of Medicine, introduced bedside teaching. All doctors today go to the bedside to learn. Osler would take medical mysteries to the laboratory to answer the questions. Halsted would take this same approach to surgical questions. For Halsted, not only the far away building with test tubes was the laboratory, but the anatomy dissecting room, and the operating room were "laboratories of the highest order". Research solved the questions raised by patient care, and research results were brought back to improve patient care.

John Staige Davis graduated in the first class from the new Johns Hopkins School of Medicine. Being among the top 12 in his class, he was chosen for the residency program at Johns Hopkins Hospital. Halsted and Osler were his teachers. Davis became interested in techniques to solve difficult wound healing problems. In 1919, Davis wrote what is considered to be the first textbook of Plastic Surgery in the United States, *Plastic Surgery: Its Principles and Practice*. The book was 770 pages long, and contained 864 illustrations and 1634 figures. This book established the specialty of Plastic Surgery in America. His wonderful biography was written by his son Bowdoin Davis, MD, who became a Plastic Surgeon.*

For the past 15 years (1993-2007) the Johns Hopkins Hospital has been ranked by U.S. World & News Reports as the number ONE hospital in the United States of America.

The first full Professor of Plastic Surgery at Johns Hopkins University and Hospital was Milton T. Edgerton, MD. He was there when I began my research at Hopkins in medical school. John E. Hoopes, MD was the second full Professor of Plastic Surgery at Johns Hopkins, and it was with him that I did my Plastic Surgery training and first research on cleft palate speech. Paul N. Manson, MD and I were Chief Residents together at Hopkins in 1978.

---

*Davis, B.W., The Life of John Staige Davis, MD, Plastic & Reconstructive Surgery, 62:368-378, 1978.

Today Dr. Manson is the Chief of Plastic Surgery at Johns Hopkins and its third full Professor of Plastic Surgery. I am just the fourth person to be a full Professor of Plastic Surgery at Johns Hopkins.

As a doctor, I am in private practice. I do not receive a salary from Johns Hopkins Hospital or University. In 1994, I had the unique honor of being the first surgeon in private practice to be promoted to Full Professor at Johns Hopkins University and the Johns Hopkins Hospital. This promotion was based upon my contributions to understanding and treatment of peripheral nerve problems. My primary appointment is in Plastic Surgery with a secondary appointment in Neurosurgery. It is my privilege to continue the tradition of research, teaching, and patient care, the three pillars, the three life times, pioneered at Johns Hopkins Hospital and Johns Hopkins University.

In the 1993, the American Society for Peripheral Nerve was begun by a small group of Plastic Surgeons interested in establishing Peripheral Nerve Surgery as a specialty. Julia K. Terzis, MD, PhD, from Norfolk , Virginia became the first President. I became the third President of this society. In January of 2008 the American Society for Peripheral Nerve will meet again. There are now about 220 members. The membership includes Orthopedic and Neurosurgeons interested in Peripheral Nerve Surgery, and two Podiatric Foot & Ankle Surgeons, but most members are Plastic Surgeons.

In the year 2002, I introduced the first Peripheral Nerve Fellowship in the World. Ivica Ducic, MD, PhD was my first Peripheral Nerve Fellow in Baltimore. Ivan's PhD was in neuroscience, and he did his Plastic Surgery training at Georgetown. He is now on the faculty at Georgetown University. Gedge D. Rosson, MD was my second Peripheral Nerve Fellow. Gedge did his Plastic Surgery training at Johns Hopkins University, and is now on the faculty at Johns Hopkins University and continues to do his Peripheral Nerve Surgery with me. Eric H. Williams, MD was the next Peripheral Nerve Fellow. Eric went to medical school at Johns Hopkins and did his Plastic Surgery training at the University of Alabama. Dr Williams has stayed on to work with me full time in Baltimore. He also has a part-time appointment at Johns Hopkins. Ziv M. Peled, MD was the next Peripheral Nerve Fellow, and the first one to train with us in Tucson, at the Dellon Institute for Peripheral Nerve Surgery: Southwest. The Dellon Institute in Tucson opened in 2003, and is directed by Christopher T. Maloney Jr, MD. Dr Peled did his Plastic Surgery training at the Harvard Combined Plastic Surgery program. Dr. Peled will begin with me the Dellon Institute for Peripheral Nerve Surgery: Northern California, located in San Francisco in July of 2007. The Dellon Institute opened in Boston in 2004, and is directed by Virginia Hung, MD. The Dellon Institute opened in St. Louis in 2006 and is directed by Robert Hagan, MD. The locations of the Dellon Institutes and the biographies of the surgeons who work there are available on line at WWW.DELLON.COM. With my commitment to research and education, the motto for the Dellon Institutes for Peripheral Nerve Surgery® is "BEING ACADEMIC IN PRIVATE PRACTICE™"

The logo for the Dellon Institutes for Peripheral Nerve Surgery® is illustrated in Figure 11-11. It was designed in the year 1999 for the opening of the first Dellon Institute which opened at Union Memorial Hospital in Baltimore in 2000, the same hospital in which I did my Hand Surgery Fellowship in 1977.

The center of the Dellon Institutes' logo in Figure 11-11 is a large myelinated nerve fiber, the type that transmits the information about touch and

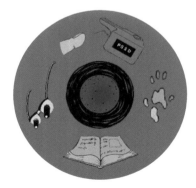

Figure 11-11. The Dellon Institutes for Peripheral Nerve Surgery® is represented by this logo.

pressure perception to the brain. The dark blue "pssd" at the top is the Pressure-Specified Sensory Device™ (which I invented with an aerospace engineer) shown measuring a fingertip's pressure threshold, representing evaluation and documentation of peripheral nerve problems. The footprint represents our basic science and clinical research. The book represents the publication of our research to inform doctors and the public about our results. The glasses are the microsurgical loupes worn in surgery to best identify and protect the nerves.

Pain is Universal and Timeless

"It is easier to find men who will volunteer to die, than to find those who are willing to endure pain with patience."

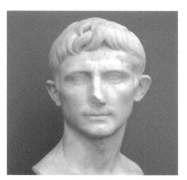

Figure 11-12. Gaius Julius Caesar, of Rome, 100 BCE.

"The greatest evil is physical pain."

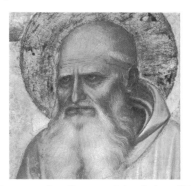

Figure 11-13. St. Augustine of Hipponemius (became island city of Tyre, coast of Palestine), 375 AD.

Why Me, and Why Now?

"Why me? Why now?" The Hopkins medical students at my lecture wanted to know. My patients want to know. I admit it seems unusual for a Plastic Surgeon to be interested in pain solutions. So where did I chose the "path less traveled"?

As I continued to investigate peripheral nerve function as a Plastic Surgeon and Hand Surgeon, I began to take care of more and more patients with pain. While most people think of neuropathy as a disease that results in numbness, ulceration and amputation of feet, about half of people with neuropathy have hand problems. For example, after I had helped a diabetic with hand problems, they would ask me if I could help their painful feet. My initial response was "no", because painful foot problems were supposedly part of a hopeless, progressive irreversible problem. Plastic Surgery is problem solving. Maybe what I did for the hands of diabetics would work for their feet. Maybe besides getting sensation back I could also get rid of chronic pain. And so I did! (See Chapter 2.)

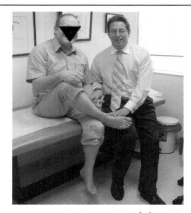

Figure 11-14. Success: one nerve, one patient at a time! A patient with diabetes who has had both legs, and then both hands operated on by me (right), decompressing multiple nerves in each extremity over the period of one year. He now has pain relief in all four extremities. His risk of developing a foot infection or having an amputation is almost gone now. His balance returns as his sensation returns.

There were other areas of pain waiting for me. As was the case with Dorothy above, my experience with cosmetic surgery (abdominoplasty) resulted in patients being referred to me to solve the groin pain puzzle. I MEASURE SUCCESS ONE PATIENT AT A TIME. The patient in Figure 11-15 is an example of this for the topic of groin pain (see Chapter 4).

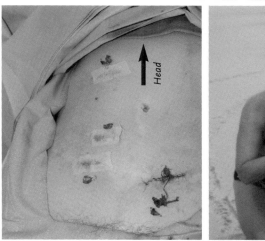 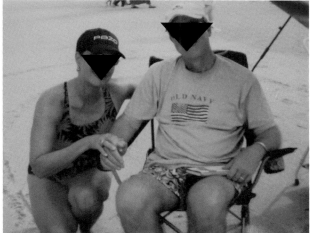

Figure 11-15. Left: Abdominal wall with direction of head noted by arrow. Sutures, Clips, Staples lie on skin after I removed them from causing nerve pain. Right: Patient with her husband, relaxing at beach 3 months after surgery. Pain relieved.

Remember that my first research in medical school involved a muscle related to speech? I began to think about nerves in the face and how they might cause pain. My newest area of work involves treatment of facial pain. This is detailed in Chapter 9. One aspect of pain is the effect is has on your daily life. I often ask patients who are troubled by pain, and especially when the recovery process from my surgery may take many months, to keep a pain diary. I ask the patient to write in blue when they are having a good day.

Pain diaries are a method of tracking improvement following surgery.

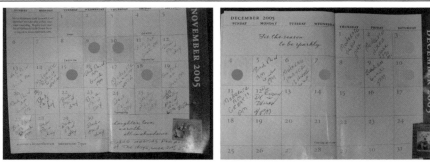

Figure 11-16. Pain diaries of patient in Figure 11-17. Her story is told in Chapter 9. The month of the left is November of 2005. There are just 4 blue dots among 30 days. The month on the right, December of 2005, has 5 blue dots among the first 11 days. She returned to see me with these diaries on December 12 to tell me she knew her pain was headed in the right direction now. For each patient, success over pain is one day at a time.

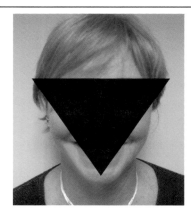

Figure 11-17. Six months since neurolysis of the right infra-orbital nerve to relieve pain in her right upper lip, cheek, and right side of her nose. She relates how she has just come back from a trip to the Southwestern U.S.A., where she was able to climb a mountain and play golf again without distracting facial pain.

I MEASURE SUCCESS ONE PATIENT AT A TIME. To achieve success for this patient meant identifying a particular sensory nerve in the face using a computer that I developed, the Pressure-Specified Sensory Device™ (more in Chapter 1 on neurosensory testing), and, borrowing from surgical techniques developed for compressed nerves in the hand, applying the technique of neurolysis to this sensory nerve in the face. There are many patients out there, and you might be one, with facial pain after cosmetic surgery, facial trauma, or removal of a tumor, who might benefit from the approach that was developed to help this woman.

Pain Relief: A Joint Decision

Plastic Surgery is problem solving.

"Why you, Doctor Dellon? Why now?" It is the same question.

I guess the reason that it is me is that I have been willing to make the effort to begin new investigations into the sources of pain related to peripheral nerve problems. In the year 2005, I received the Plastic Surgery Educational Foundation Prize for my work on using the Pressure-Specified Sensory Device™ (PSSD) to identify early nerve involvement in patients with Leprosy. In this new research, I applied the operations I developed to restore sensation and prevent amputation in patients with diabetes to patients with Leprosy (see Chapter 2). There are still millions of people disabled world-wide with Leprosy despite the use of antibiotics, which kill the bacteria but do not reverse the nerve damage caused by the bacteria living within the nerve. Patients with Leprosy (now called Hansen's disease) do not have joint pain, because the nerves to their joints have died, and not send pain signals. What does that suggest about the treatment of joint pain today?

In 1979, I identified the nerve to the back of the wrist joint. This occurred during removal of what I thought was a recurrent cyst, but proved to be a painful neuroma on the back of the wrist joint. This was a surprise, since no anatomy book showed a nerve to the back of the wrist joint. In fact, anatomy books do not show any nerves to joints. If there are no nerves to joints, why do so many elderly patients, so many athletes, and so many people with injuries have joint pain? (See chapter 3.) Plastic Surgery is problem solving!

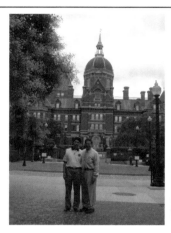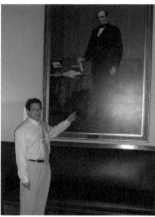

Figure 11-18. Left: Dr. Dellon with Dr. Yong Yao, a Neurosurgeon from Beijing, China standing in front of the Johns Hopkins Hospital in 2004. Right: Dr. Dellon with portrait of Mr. Johns Hopkins, the benefactor of the Johns Hopkins Hospital.

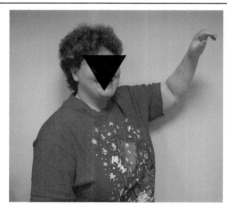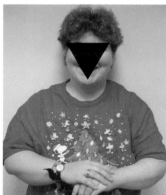

Figure 11-19. My Christmas present to this women was denervation of her left shoulder so she could lift her arm without pain again (left) and to denervate the back of her hand so she could touch it again without pain (right). She was injured 4 years previously. She is back at work teaching handicapped children. She is off all her pain medications. I MEASURE SUCCESS ONE PATIENT AT A TIME.

Following the Johns Hopkins tradition of identifying a clinical problem and taking it to the laboratory, I began what has turned out to be a new field of peripheral nerve surgery: PARTIAL JOINT DENERVATION. In 2004, I received the Plastic Surgery Educational Foundation Senior Research Award for this concept and this body of work. Specific joint pain problems are covered in Chapter 3. Here is just one example of a patient whose crushed left hand resulted in a painful wrist and a painful shoulder (see Figure 11-19).

My training at Johns Hopkins School of Medicine taught me the approach to problem solving that I have been able to apply to the treatment of pain problems. My Plastic Surgery training at Johns Hopkins Hospital gave me the surgical skills to identify and correct pain related to the peripheral nerve. In March, 2007, the University of Utrecht in Holland, awarded me a PhD (see Figure 11-20) for my work related to treating the symptoms of diabetic neuropathy. This book, *Pain Solutions,* is my current approach to the diagnosis and treatment of the most common pain problems.

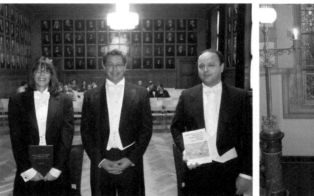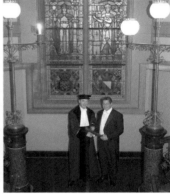

Figure 11-20. In March, 2007, Dr Dellon received a PhD for his work related to relieving the symptoms of diabetic neuropathy. On the left, he is the ancient hall of the University of Utrecht, where his Thesis Defense was held, and flanked by Luiann Greer Dellon, and Henk Coert, MD, PhD, each holding a copy of the thesis. On the right, Dr Moshe Kon, MD, PhD, Chief of Plastic Surgery at the University of Utrecht, stands with Dr Dellon.

Index

"Find a page with a
hopeful story
and a pain solution
for you here."

NOTES

OTHER BOOKS BY A. LEE DELLON

Evaluation of Sensibility and Re-Education of Sensation in the Hand

First Printing, 1981 / Second Printing, 1984 / Third Printing, 1988 / Japanese Translation, 1994

Surgery of the Peripheral Nerve

co-authored with S. E. Mackinnon

First Printing, 1989 / Second Printing, 1991 / Chinese Translation, 1991 / Japanese Translation, 1992

Somatosensory Testing and Rehabilitation

First Printing, 1997 / Second Printing, 2000

Interpretation Guide to Neurosensory and Motor Testing

co-authored with D. K. Seiler and S.L. Barrett

First Printing, 2002

Surgical Approach to Lower Extremity Nerve Decompression in the Patient with Diabetic Neuropathy

First Printing, 2006

Interpretation Guide to Neurosensory and Motor Testing: the PDA Platform

co-authored with D. K. Seiler and L. Motwani

First Printing, 2007